Christmas 1986
To Mary
with all my love
John xxx

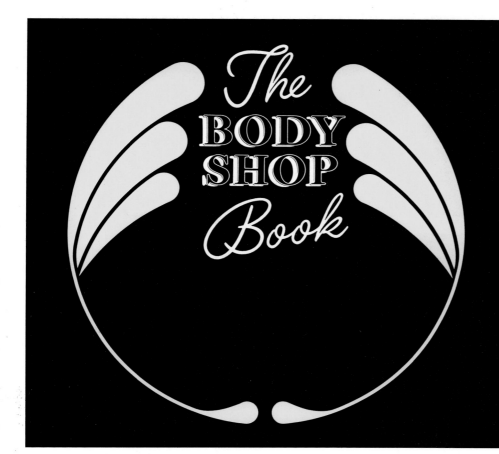

The BODY SHOP Book

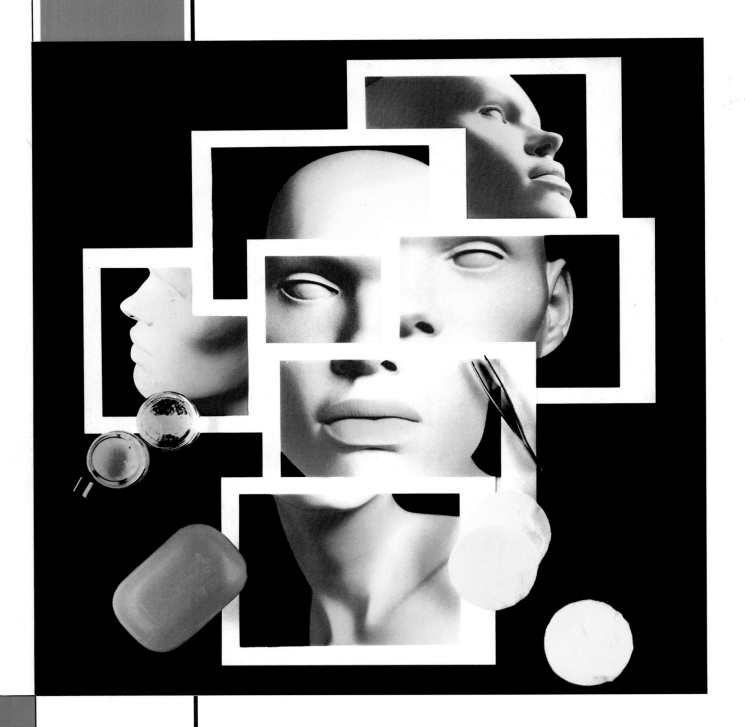

The **BODY SHOP** *Book*

FOREWORD BY ANITA RODDICK

Macdonald

A **Macdonald** BOOK

Text © The Body Shop International plc 1985
Design & illustration © Shuckburgh Reynolds Ltd 1985

First published in Great Britain in 1985
by Macdonald & Co (Publishers) Ltd
London & Sydney
A member of BPCC plc
Reprinted 1986

Produced, edited and designed by
Shuckburgh Reynolds Ltd
289 Westbourne Grove, London W11 2QA

British Library Cataloguing in Publication Data
The Body shop book.
  1. Beauty, Personal
  I. Roddick, Anita
  646.7'2   RA776.98

ISBN 0-356-10934-8

Typeset by SX Composing Ltd, Rayleigh, Essex

Printed and bound in Spain by
Printer Industria Grafica SA, Barcelona, DLB 231 89/85

Macdonald & Co (Publishers) Ltd
Maxwell House
74 Worship Street, London EC2A 2EN

CONTENTS

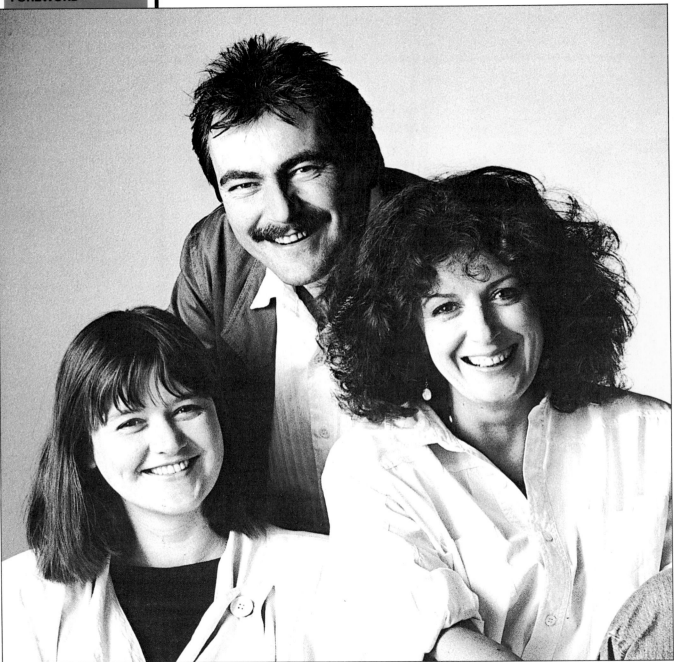

FOREWORD

I N 1976 I OPENED THE BODY SHOP IN A BACK STREET IN BRIGHTON. With £4000 borrowed from the bank I could only afford to spend £700 on products, but the 20 products we formulated looked pretty pathetic all standing on one shelf, so to make the shop look busy and full I produced them in five sizes of bottle. I couldn't afford fancy packaging so I bought the cheapest bottles available and the labels were handwritten. We painted the ceiling of our tiny shop green to cover the damp patches and put garden fencing on the walls to stop the rain splashing the products. The first day we opened was a Saturday and we took £100. The other retailers in the street were laying odds of 10-1 against our surviving six months, but we were on our way.

The idea of The Body Shop is not new. In India and the Arab world for centuries perfume has been decanted and sold in the amounts the customer wanted, and in California in the sixties you could bring your own bottle and get it filled. Greengrocers and confectioners also trade in this way: you can buy as much or as little as you want. What was new was that we applied it to cosmetics. And unintentionally, due to lack of money, we produced these other individual features which, apart from the handwritten labels, will always be with us.

The ideas for the products were based on my experiences travelling around the world. I saw raw ingredients being used, as they had been for centuries, to polish the skin, to cleanse the hair and to protect both. They worked, without hype, without claims and without millions spent on advertising. And they were and still are the building blocks from which all our products are created.

The cosmetics industry today is dominated by men, who use fear to create needs women don't have, and sell them camouflage under the heading 'beauty'. Make no mistake, these men are talking to themselves, not to women. One of my greatest pleasures in running The Body Shop is the tremendous input of women, who own and run more than 90 per cent of our shops. We feel the word 'beauty' is old-fashioned and ally ourselves strongly with health and lifestyle. We also feel it is healthy to question the role of cosmetics in society. Our customers ask us increasingly discerning questions and we believe we have an obligation to respond to their needs and give them the information they want.

The production of this book was an amazing experience which could never have been achieved without the help of all the contributors, but in particular I have enjoyed the close co-operation of Mark Constantine, our herbalist, who has never flagged in his enthusiasm for the project and Deb McCormick, who has probed and prodded every statement. After seemingly endless discussion and argument our beliefs are as strong now as they were when we started, and I would like to thank them both.

Anita Roddick

Opposite, *from left to right: Deb McCormick, Mark Constantine and Anita Roddick.*

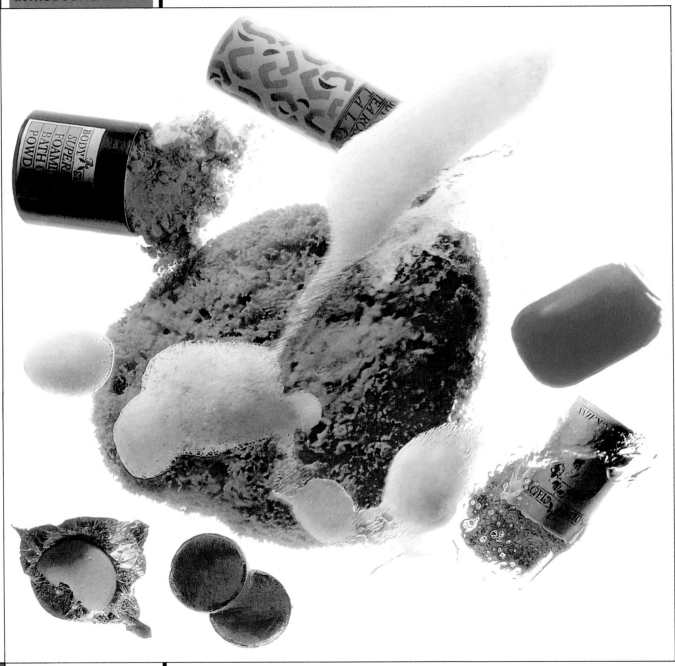

THE BODY SHOP

AN IDEA WHOSE TIME HAS COME

BEFORE 1976, WHEN THE FIRST BODY SHOP OPENED IN BRIGHTON, there was something intimidating about buying cosmetics. They were usually sold by heavily made-up staff from behind gleaming counters. They came lavishly wrapped and were often available in one size only. When you undid the cellophane, ribbon and box, and threw them straight in the bin, you had already thrown away most of your money (packaging would account for about 85% of the price) and if you then found you did not like the product you had wasted the rest.

Many of the basic features of the Body Shop came about through a combination of necessity and happy accident. Anita Roddick wanted to buy her cosmetics in the same way she bought her groceries — as much or as little as she wanted. When she began to sell her own cosmetics, she therefore introduced five sizes of bottle, enabling customers to invest less than one pound before they decided whether they liked the product. Financial necessity dictated that the bottles were the cheapest available, but it was a happy accident that she ran out of them in her first week of business. She then suggested to her customers that they bring back their bottles to be refilled — and so one of the unique features of the Body Shop, the Refill Bar, was born. Many other positive aspects of the business resulted from an initial lack of financial resources. Big-budget advertising and expensive packaging were out of the question, but this in turn meant that the products could be sold inexpensively without sacrificing quality. As word got round and the range became successful all the profits could be used to explore new ideas and devise more products. Without the heavy financial commitment of advertising and fancy packaging the Body Shop was free to try out new ideas and assimilate the knowledge quickly. This flexibility soon became one of its greatest strengths.

Limited finance was also the reason why the business was extended by franchise, which again had a positive effect. The owners of the franchises were highly involved in the company and helped to maintain its energy. Ideas and information were pooled in the interest of all concerned and channels of communication were kept constantly open. This direct access to the company encouraged the flow of ideas, and the fact that these ideas were then tried out in turn stimulated more. It is for this reason that we now have the most extensive range of skin and hair care products in this country.

WHERE OUR IDEAS COME FROM

Education is the cornerstone on which the future of the Body Shop rests. It is essential for us to pursue new discoveries and unearth the knowledge of the past which has been lost by our modern technological society. Constant travel enables us to learn from the cultural traditions handed down from generation to generation among different peoples of the world. When she was travelling in Mexico, for

Throughout this book you will find snippets of useful information introduced by the following signs:

This sign means **Fact:** statistics, myth-breakers or simply interesting pieces of information are introduced by it.

The triangle denotes a **Warning:** read these carefully to protect yourself from harm.

A circle introduces a **Tip:** recipes, hints and DIY health tips.

example, Anita Roddick observed that aloe plants were kept in the home; if there was an accident in which someone was burnt, an aloe leaf was broken off and its gel applied directly to the wound. In less sophisticated societies than our own, raw ingredients are still used automatically in the treatment of skin and hair problems. In the West we have forgotten this knowledge and reach automatically for a proprietary brand of medicine which advertisements have assured us will cure all our problems.

In the Body Shop raw ingredients are the building blocks of our cosmetic preparations. When Anita watched the Polynesians scoop up untreated cocoa butter and apply it direct to their skin and then felt the smooth texture of the skin, she determined that cocoa butter would be an important ingredient in our skin care products. From Sri Lanka she learned that people there use pineapple as a skin cleanser and on returning home she looked into the scientific basis for this tradition. Washington's Library of Medicine collates information of pharmaceutical and cosmetic interest from 110 countries around the world and from them she learned that the natural enzymes present in pineapple act on the skin to remove dead cells, making it an effective skin cleanser.

It is this marriage of traditional wisdom and knowledge of raw ingredients with modern scientific research that makes Body Shop products unique and effective. We are in constant touch with the Library of Medicine and are amongst the first to hear of any new discoveries relating to cosmetic ingredients. However, to date we have been proved correct in our thesis that nothing can nourish the skin when applied to the surface and nothing can rejuvenate it. Skin care is about prevention. And prevention is about cleansing, exfoliating and protection.

THE BODY SHOP PHILOSOPHY

Body Shop products are natural, biodegradable and are prepared without cruelty to animals. There are also some aspects of the cosmetic industry which we believe are unpalatable:

* Animals should not suffer in laboratory tests for our vanity
* Whales should not be slaughtered to provide moisture creams
* Placenta is unacceptable as a cosmetic ingredient
* Aerosols should not be used as they are indisposable and damage the environment
* Packaging should not be wasteful or unnecessarily expensive

ANIMAL EXPERIMENTS

The first experiment to test cosmetics by squirting substances into the eyes of animals was conducted in 1941 and three years later J. H. Draize described the basic technique, which was conducted on rabbits. One eye was left untouched, as a control, and the other was squirted with the chosen substance. The eyes were rinsed at varying intervals and the level of eye irritation given a score by the researcher. The experiment has since become common practice and is known as the Draize Test.

The other widely used test in the cosmetics industry is known as the LD50 Test and involves feeding chemicals to a group of animals. The researcher records how much of the substance can be eaten before causing death to half the animals.

Even if you could ignore the cruelty involved in these tests, it is difficult to ignore the lack of scientific precision. In the Draize Test, the severity of irritation is a subjective measure and one laboratory technician's idea of a grade 2 injury might be another's grade 4. The unreliability of the test has been further shown by other unpalatable research, which has proved that rabbits' eyes are quite different from those of hamsters, dogs, rats, monkeys and guinea pigs. The atypical nature of a rabbit's eye was also shown by another experiment which tested shampoos which were already on the market. Although these products had a troublefree sales history they caused irritation when tested on rabbits' eyes.

The crudeness of the LD50 Test can be judged by the difference in size between humans and guinea pigs, on which the test is usually performed. It is also well known that extreme doses of any substance can be fatal. **If these tests are useless, why do they continue to be used**?

The pressure brought to bear by the general public and the success of companies like the Body Shop have succeeded in reducing the use of these cruel tests. The Fund for the Replacement of Animals in Medical Experiments (FRAME) hopes that their use will cease entirely by 1988. This, however, remains to be seen. In 1984, 2500 rabbits were subjected to the Draize Test and many more were used in other tests on raw materials for the cosmetic industry.

A large number of these tests were conducted for cosmetics that had already been used satisfactorily for some time in many countries. Japan in particular, but also Israel, Mexico and Holland insisted on doing animal tests before they would accept the products for their markets. Why? The only possible answer is a form of restrictive practice, to protect their own manufacturers and force competitors into long unnecessary tests to keep them out of their domestic market.

SAFETY WITHOUT ANIMAL TESTING

Experiments on animals are not necessary to ensure that a product is safe. Making cosmetics is rather like cookery, in that both have been practised and refined for thousands of years. At some time almost anything which might be a source of food has been tried and by trial and error people have found the most useful ingredients and discovered the best ways to combine them. Similarly, people in every part of the world have used the natural products of their environment to enhance their bodies and have discovered which are the most effective.

We have inherited a wealth of practical knowledge of raw ingredients. And just as flour, eggs and water can be combined in various ways to make many different cakes, so we know that simple raw ingredients such as cocoa butter, almond oil and water can be made into many different cosmetics. By using the raw ingredients which have this long history of safe and effective use, we can be assured of the safety of the products.

Hair dyes are a good example. For over 5000 years, henna and indigo have been in use and for 3000 of these years their use has been documented. There must be very little that they can do to the hair or body that would not have been noticed in this time and the only known side-effect is that indigo causes some people who are prone to allergies to sneeze if they sniff it. Synthetic hair dyes, on the other hand, have only about 80 years of history and in that short time they have caused many problems, not least in their suspected links with cancer.

If a product is developed from ingredients which are known to be safe it can be tested on people. This also has the great advantage that people can tell you what they

Fact: unpalatable
Edible snails have been used in cosmetics and medicines for thousands of years. Galen devoted a chapter to them in his medical treatise; Italian and French peasants have used them for centuries. Tests carried out in 1960 on homogenized snails in creams and face packs proved them to be effective, if inhumane, moisturizers.

Fact: unreliable
A comparative EEC study into the notorious LD50 animal test has shown that the results of this experiment varied by a factor of eight between different laboratories when testing the same material.

think of the product and express any reservations at the testing stage. We use independent volunteers, many of them Animal Aid supporters, who test the products by using them normally and then describing their effects. To test new synthetic ingredients the *in vitro* test, developed by Dr Bruce Ames of California University, can be used. This involves breeding cell cultures in the laboratory and then studying the effects on them of different chemical solutions. Apart from the obvious advantage of not being cruel to animals this test is also far more sophisticated and reliable.

"NATURAL" COSMETICS

The label "natural cosmetics" has a distinct meaning for us. We use ingredients as close to their natural source as possible; we conduct no animal experiments and we ensure that our cosmetics cause no harm to anyone or anything in their production. However, it is not enough for the products to be pure. They must also be effective. We therefore accept the need to add a percentage of synthetic preservative, provided it has not been tested on animals, in order to protect the product from deterioration.

Oils used in the production of our cosmetics are bought raw and cold pressed to ensure that their efficacy has not been affected by refining. Similarly, we check that the essential qualities of the herbs used in our products are not diminished by poor extraction methods. Many of our ingredients, such as glycerine, can be obtained either from an animal or a vegetable source, in which case we always use the vegetable source. Where there is this choice, we see no reason why animals should be killed to provide cosmetic ingredients. We try to ensure that every element in a Body Shop product is there for a purpose. For example, the perfume in the products is provided by essential oils which are beneficial to the skin as well as pleasant to smell.

PRESERVATIVES

A common concern about natural cosmetics is that they will deteriorate quickly as a result of bacterial activity. The EEC requires the inclusion of a certain amount of preservative and we use two of the safest available – methyl and propilparaban – both of which occur naturally in B vitamins. We also employ independent microbiologists to screen our products.

We are concerned by the cosmetic industry's use of high levels of preservatives, which can be toxic and may also damage the fine balance of beneficial bacteria present. Some harsh anti-bacterial creams, for example, destroy the bacteria present and may leave opportunities for more harmful bacteria to replace them, just as over-medication for minor illnesses can leave the body vulnerable to attacks from more virulent complaints.

THE ENVIRONMENT

We believe in conducting our business without causing harm to the environment. Our products are biodegradable and can safely be washed down the plug-hole along with the bath water without fear of them building up indestructable residues in the earth and destroying the ecological balance.

As David Bellamy has said, we cannot keep taking from the earth without destroying the balance essential to life. We try to avoid wastes of natural resources by keeping our packaging simple and encouraging our customers to re-use their bottles at our Refill Bar. As well as minimizing waste this also helps to keep prices down. If the product is bought as a gift the customer can wrap it, but if it is for personal use nobody has to pay for unnecessary wrapping.

We operate the same policy at our manufacturing and distribution plants, recycling cardboard containers and even using packing protections for decoration in our gift packs. We are planning to employ a waste officer to examine alternatives to our operations with a view to cutting down even further on our waste.

PUTTING IDEAS INTO PRACTICE

The easiest way to see how our cosmetics are produced is to follow the development of one product from initial idea to finished item. In this case the product is our Honeyed Beeswax and Almond Oil Cleanser. Our intention was to produce an effective cleanser which would leave the skin clean and would be suitable both for dry and sensitive skins.

Our first step was to do some historical research. The earliest written record of a cleansing cream was by the Greek physician Galen in his *Methodus Medendi Vel de Marbis Curandis*, in the second century AD. He described a mixture of beeswax, oil and rosewater, the first time a combination of oils and water had been suggested. It was such a success that this mixture formed the basis for cold creams and cleansing creams until very recently.

Changes were made to this formula because, to quote the cosmetic industry's handbook Harry, "by modern standards none (of the ingredients) would be acceptable due to instability, poor appearance and poor reproduceability of manufacture". In the eighteenth century spermaceti, a waxy substance obtained from sperm whales, was added to produce a lighter cream. Before 1900 mineral oil replaced the vegetable oil — "the primary object of the substitution being to ensure whiteness, inhibition of rancidity and uniformity of finished product" (Harry).

Today, cleansing creams are made from many different synthetic ingredients: no rosewater and very seldom beeswax or vegetable oil. None of these changes to the original formula had anything to do with the mixture's effect on the skin. They were introduced to make the product look more attractive in the pot and to make it easier and cheaper to produce.

Our next step was to do some practical research. We found that in comparative tests on the skin the original Galen formula was excellent. If removed properly with cotton wool dipped in warm water it was more effective than any modern cream. We produced a cleanser with almond oil, beeswax and honey (from our own hives) and rosewater. It was a loose emulsion with brown bits from the bees' dirty feet! A year later we managed to produce a lighter, creamier version using a homogeniser, and we strained out the bees' footprints. We then added preservatives to give the product a long shelf life and to abide by the new EEC regulations. Later, we decided to add jojoba oil, the vegetable equivalent of spermaceti. This made the product easier to apply and left the skin softer.

Three years after our initial research we started trials using honeyed beeswax on acne and sensitive skins. The trials proved successful and the product was ready to go on sale. We are now successfully selling a formula which is little different from the one described nearly 2000 years ago.

Did you know?
In 1974, 478 million aerosols were sold in the UK, approximately eight per person. Aerosol containers are made of a high grade metal which is a rare resource and yet it cannot be recycled.

Tip: from Mintel study
One of the findings of this British research project was that the colour of foundation creams can alter on oily skins. Change to a foundation formulated specifically for oily skin, and test it in natural light.

FUTURE BOTANICALS

As the demand for natural cosmetics increases, so does research into herbs and natural oils, and consequently we now have many new and exciting raw materials to experiment with. Camellia or tsubaki oil is produced from a Japanese evergreen plant whose seeds are pressed for the light, sweet oil. It gives shine to the hair and is emollient on the skin, so we are testing it in hairdressings and massage oils.

Orizaoil is another interesting Oriental oil, made from rice seed, which may enable us to "fix" colours to prevent them fading. It could then be used to produce natural lipsticks and eye shadows and would make a good base for creams. Shea butter, a fat produced from an African nut, is traditionally used in Ghana as an emollient for the skin. It has proved especially useful for protecting the skin from the wear and tear of city pollution.

The Body Shop has spent years evaluating other plants which are already in use cosmetically. As an example, we have been testing the supposed miracle powers of the Evening Primrose for the last few years. Many claims made for this plant, traditionally known as The King's Cure-all, would appear to be wishful thinking, but others are very exciting.

As the dangers of sun tanning become more widely known, research is being conducted into the use of herbs to protect the skin from the sun. One of the most effective is carrot oil, which we already use for its cosmetic effects and will be using increasingly to develop new products. Mustard oil has been used for hundreds of years in Pakistan, India and Arabia and its ability to aid the creation of Vitamin D in the skin makes it unique. This also works especially well in sunny conditions to help dry, flaky skin. Add to these items as varied as pumpkin seed oil, yeast, walnut kernels and strawberry enzymes and you get an idea of the further potential of using botanical raw materials.

WHERE DO WE GO FROM HERE?

It is often assumed that success is the end of the story. For us it is just the beginning. It means that we have got to work harder to stay out in front, to come up with more original ideas - but it also means that we have more resources to develop our ideas.

One idea we are currently working on is a massage school. We are particularly interested in the therapeutic effects of massage and would like to see qualified masseurs in hospitals, especially in geriatric and in psychiatric wards. We hope eventually to be able to supply some of these masseurs, as we believe that massage is an effective treatment for long stay patients and can contribute to making their lives happier and healthier. We would also like to work with the parents of young children, teaching them how to massage their babies — a soothing skill that has been forgotten in our modern society.

Another project close to our hearts is the Education Pack that we are working on. Our aim is to provide an interesting and informative teaching aid from which children can learn how cosmetics are made, where the ingredients come from and how they work. We would also like to encourage them to consider aspects of retailing. Shopping is a regular part of our daily lives which is often taken for granted and we think it is important to know how the retail trade operates. If we can encourage children to look objectively at their High Streets perhaps we will see higher standards in the future.

One aspect of retailing which we should like to see questioned is that of design. Shopping is increasingly a leisure activity and as such should be pleasurable. We hope that by making children aware of shops as an important feature in their environment, the next generation will take more care to question architectural decisions which have a permanent effect on the landscape. We would also like to make children aware of shop displays and understand how they work in terms of colour, structure and volume. Shop display is a form of street theatre and if we can make children see it as such they will find retailing exciting. We are, after all, a nation of shopkeepers! Shops have rested on their laurels for too long and, as each and every one of us uses shops, we should demand higher standards of service.

Success does not make life easy. We have always encouraged our customers to let us know their opinions of our products and they do! For instance, if someone finds they have an allergy to a product they tell us. We work out what may have caused the allergic reaction and inform our herbalists and chemists who keep data on all the products. We also check our Product Information File for other products containing the sensitizing ingredient so that the customer can find an alternative. We would like to see this kind of service become common practice in all shops. You should be able to get good advice about anything you buy from the place you bought it. Only by constantly asking for advice and expecting sales assistance will we make our shops the places we want them to be. The day of uninterested, uninformed and unhappy sales staff is over.

HOW THE SHOPS WORK

The first time you enter a Body Shop can be confusing as you are confronted by shelf upon shelf of coloured bottles and row upon row of creams. To help you choose the right product for yourself we have a three-tiered information system.

Firstly, the labels explain who the product is suitable for, how to use it and what significant properties it has. If you would like to know more there is a Product Information File available on the counter. This is particularly useful for customers with allergy problems as they can check for their sensitizing ingredient and avoid those products that contain it. Secondly, the sales staff are trained to know technical information about skin and hair and about the products. We do not teach the staff sales tricks because we believe that if someone is given the correct information and chooses the right product then the product will sell itself. Neither do we indulge in gimmicks to encourage sales, because we would prefer you to pay for what you want rather than for useless "free" gifts.

If, exceptionally, our staff cannot deal with your queries our final tier of information is the herbalists or cosmetic chemists who created the products, to whom we have immediate access. This ability to communicate directly ensures that the chemists and herbalists have practical information and the latest research to help them develop their ideas. Many respected chemists in the cosmetic industry are dismayed when they see what happens to the products they have created once they leave the laboratory. Products designed for one purpose are often loaded with advertising claims that promise the impossible.

THE BODY SHOP BOOK

We have set out this book like a Body Shop walkabout. Each section of the book

Fact: cosmetics
At any given time, the average consumer is using between 11 and 12 cosmetic products.

Fact: and fiction
"Hope is what we sell in cosmetics" *(The Toilet Goods Association)*

Fact: cosmetic junk
Many women's dressing tables are cluttered with "dead enthusiasm" – stale jars, unopened bottles, half-used boxes of cosmetics.

Fact: healing aloe
The healing powers of aloe first came to the attention of the U.S. Government when it was shown that Japanese victims of atomic radiation who were treated with aloe gel healed more quickly.

Fact: skin deep
You shed 100 million skin particles every two and a half minutes and inhale large amounts of them with every deep breath. Statistically, you could inhale the complete covering of a person's skin in the time it takes to follow 600 people up the escalator at Holborn Tube station.

represents an area of the shop and the information from our three-tier system is distilled to help you to choose from the options available and to explain why we have adopted the stances we do.

This is not a beauty book. We have taken the word "beauty" out of our vocabulary because we believe it encourages false dreams. The Body Shop is not in the beauty business. You will find no real faces in this book because the cosmetics industry uses glossy advertisements to sell miracle answers: "Use this cream and you will look like this." You won't. Behind each photograph of a flawless 20-year-old advertising a rejuvenating cream is a team of dream-makers: the make-up artist painting out the blemishes, the hair stylist constantly adjusting the hair and the photographer lighting and retouching the image. Even the models don't look like this in real life.

We do not want to feed the dissatisfaction that is bred by these unattainable dreams. Beautiful women have long been used to endorse cosmetic remedies. In the past you might have been told that you too could look like Helen of Troy or Cleopatra if you used this preparation. But it was the advent of the film industry which provided glamorous heroines and fuelled the desire for personal beauty. If you looked like Hedy Lamarr, you too would be carried off into the sunset. Life would be so much better and you would be so much happier if only you were more beautiful. The movie moguls fed off this desire and stage-managed their stars'.lives so that they were never seen without the studio stamp of glamour, packaged into confections of powder and bleached hair.

We do not believe in encouraging these false images of beauty. Even the stars themselves or the photographic models do not see their own beauty, only a two-dimensional graphic or celluloid version of what someone else thinks beauty should be. We prefer to work with reality, and in this book we would like to show you:

* How to look after and enjoy your body
* How to avoid damaging your skin and hair
* How to make the most of what you've got
* All the hidden issues behind the cosmetics industry
* Tricks and treats of the trade

But finally it is about options. **Here is the information. You make the choice**.

HAIR

WHAT IS HAIR?

HAIR CARE

HAIR PROBLEMS

HAIR COLOUR

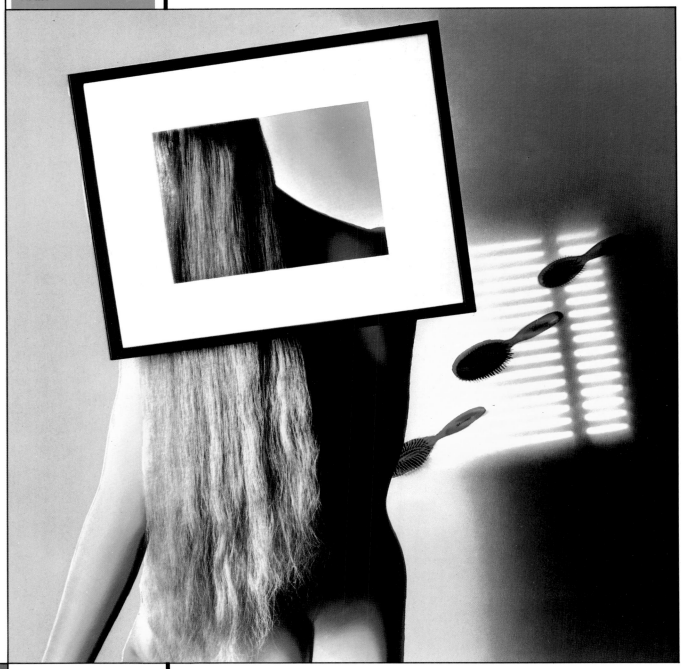

WHAT IS HAIR?

ALL THOSE WASTED PAINS ON ARRANGING YOUR HAIR – WHAT contribution can it make to your salvation? One minute you are building it up and the next you are letting it down . . . Some women spend all their energy forcing their hair to curl, others make it look loose and wavy, in a style that may look natural but is not natural at all."

So said Tertullian, the Carthaginian theologian, in the second century, and women's attitude to hair has barely changed since then.

According to some psychologists, hair is the first thing we notice about a person. It has sexual connotations and while we, initially, keep our primary sexual characteristics under wraps, the hair becomes a secondary focus of our sexuality. Because it is both decorative and versatile we can choose the image we want to project at any given time. We can cut it, colour it, twist it or plait it, sweep it up, hide behind it or, ultimately, shave the lot off. No other part of our body has such incredible flexibility. Hair is fascinating stuff, a glorious material to play with and enjoy.

The 18th century excelled at outlandish hairdos: men still wore wigs, and the women, anxious to assert their difference, built up competitively elaborate styles with the help of pads made from pigs' hair, and extra hairpieces. Some of the court beauties had more need of structural engineers than maids to do their hair. Horace Walpole was reprimanded for smirking at the sight of one recently married lady's hairstyle: "She came out one night to Northumberland House with such a display of frizz that it literally spread beyond her shoulders. I happened to say that it looked as if her parents had stinted her in hair before her marriage and that she is determined to indulge her fancy now".

Posterity will no doubt comment upon the late 20th century's innovative punk styles and debate the use of hair as a lethal weapon from the superglue that was employed to keep the hair in dangerously rigid spikes. It must, though, be regarded as some kind of progress that women's hair is no longer used as a convenient dishcloth the way it sometimes was in earlier centuries.

Great emotional associations centre around hair: men mourn its loss and pay through the nose for transplants; women chop off their hair as they change lovers or jobs; and tears are shed over the first ringlet cut from a baby's hair. It has been woven into eternity rings – hair takes longer than flesh to disintegrate and perhaps lasts longer than feelings. If you wanted to, you could probably knit a durable jumper from human hair.

THE PURPOSE OF HAIR

The whole body is covered with hairs with the exception of the lips, the soles of the feet and the palms of the hand. On the body, the hair, called vellous hair, is fine and downy, more so on the female body, while the hair of eyelashes, eyebrows and nostrils is coarser because it is designed to protect the sensitive eyes and nose from

The price of beauty
Wigs were rich spoils in the 18th century when they could fetch up to 50 guineas on the black market. Children, secreted in large baskets on the shoulders of would-be muggers, would reach out as carriages passed and snatch the wigs.

Danger: pains for beauty
One monumental hair style chosen by an 18th century courtier proved fatal: the lady brushed past a chandelier, the mass of wool and grease in her hairdo caught fire, and she died of burns.

Opposite: *hair is beautiful. Long or short, straight or curly, it responds to loving care with shine and vitality. It echoes our every mood, mirrors our dreams and hidden fantasies.*

Opposite: *the miracle of hair is the way it grows, squeezing its way through minute follicles like paste through a tube. Hereditary genes determine the thickness of each single hair, and nothing can transform a coarse mane into baby-fine wisps. Genes are also responsible for the hair's shape, but this can be changed with perms and straighteners.*

irritation and to prevent entry of bacteria and germs. Underarm and pubic hair is generally longer and softer, possibly because its purpose is to prevent chafing of sensitive skin areas, though it is also useful to have longer hair to allow sweat a route through to the air. Sweat serves to cool the body, and does so marvellously, though it has a less marvellous odour when it's been around for a while.

The hair on the scalp grows the longest and thickest and helps to protect the brain, that most sensitive organ. It is the crowning head hair that requires the most meticulous attention, although body hair also needs personal hygiene.

THE STRUCTURE OF HAIR

Hair is incredibly strong, even stronger than copper wire of the same thickness. It consists of three layers: the cuticle, which is the outside layer of overlapping scales, invisible because the layer is transparent; the cortex, composed of cells which provide stretch and strength and which also contain the colour pigment that shows through the transparent cuticles; and the medulla, the innermost core of each hair, formed of round cells which give thickness to the hair shaft, and which is sometimes missing in fine hair. The medulla was once thought to be a canal for a life-giving fluid, a belief which resulted in the peculiar practice of singeing split ends in order to staunch the flow of this fluid. This is nonsense; no fluid runs down the shaft of the hair, and each visible hair is in effect dead.

HOW HAIR GROWS

Imagine a tube of toothpaste: squeezing the paste out of the tube is similar to the way hair is pushed through the skin from its origin of growth, the follicle. Every single hair starts from a follicle, and the larger the follicle, the thicker the hair. This is unchangeable. If the follicle sits vertically in the scalp you will have straight hair; if it is bent or curved you will have curly or wavy hair. This *is* changeable as perms and straighteners can be used to undo what the follicle intended, and as soon as a hair emerges from the scalp, chemicals attack and weaken it, causing structural changes. Beneath each hair follicle is a small muscle, the erector muscle, which contracts and causes the hair to stand on end when you are cold or frightened. The function of these muscles is more obvious in animals, and is very inconspicuous in humans.

Attached to each follicle are sebaceous gland sacs which pump out sebum, the hair's lubricant oil. The impetus of the production line comes from a clump of cells, the papillae, at the base of the follicle. Fed by capillaries they become engorged with blood and are stimulated to produce hair cells; as these cells harden (keratinize) and die, they become the hair shaft.

Hair has one of the most prolific growth rates in the whole body and is at its most productive between the ages of 11-30. It passes through three distinct phases, after which it stays unproductive for approximately three months and then usually starts all over again. However, if the capillaries are constricted or the papilla itself is damaged or programmed to desist, it cannot generate replacement hair. Growth is determined by genetic factors which dictate that men more often than women will be unable to produce replacement hair. Recent evidence would suggest that women who have demanding and competitive careers run an increased risk of hair loss.

The anogen phase is the first and beneficial phase of the growth cycle. The papilla is fed constantly and produces hair cells which push out hair at the rate of

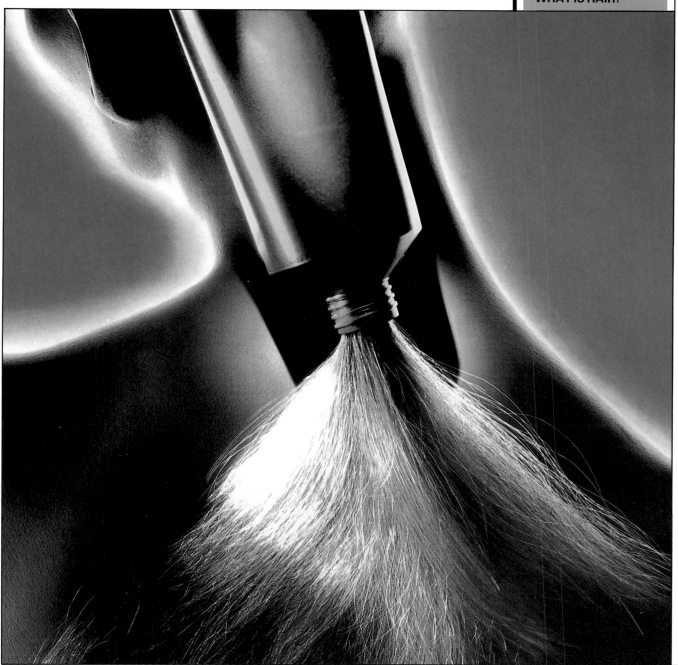

Tip: from the horse's mouth
Take a tip from the vet;
vitamin B supplements
improve the coats of
animals and work wonders
for human hair.

approximately 12 mm per month. At any given time about 85% of hair is at this stage of development; the phase can last from two to seven years and determines how long your hair will grow. During the second stage, **the telogen phase,** keratinization ceases, and a kind of holding operation commences which lasts for a mere few weeks before the final phase, **the catogen phase.** This isn't as much a phase as the termination of growth. The hair falls out. At this stage you might panic. Standing dripping over the sink, you notice a couple of loose hairs. You start to pull them out of the plug hole only to be confronted with a nasty little sausage of hairs. Calm down. It is quite **normal** to lose between 50-150 hairs every day, and more during hormonal upheavals such as menstruation, pregnancy and the menopause. For your hair to show as thinning you would have to lose between 40-50% from one area.

Everyone is born with a finite number of hair follicles which remains static. An average count would reveal between 90,000-150,000 or more hairs per head. Blondes have the largest number of follicles, usually because they have the finest hair; brunettes are average, and redheads have the least. Paradoxically, redheads *appear* to have the most abundant hair because their hair follicles are larger and their hair is therefore thicker.

WHAT AFFECTS HAIR?

Egyptian mummies have been unwrapped to reveal hair that has been preserved for centuries. Why then do we now have such problems with brittle and damaged hair?

Environmental influences
*leave their marks: grime-
laden rain, pool-water
chemicals and adulterated
tap water dull and deaden
the hair as surely as
shampoo left unrinsed. The
lack of air moisture in our
centrally heated homes
dries and snarls the hair as
effectively as a strong
autumn gale (far right).*

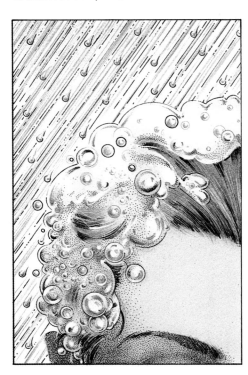

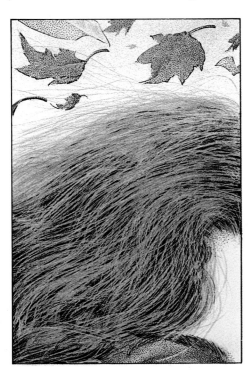

In more than 75% of cases the damage is self-inflicted. We are our hair's worst enemies. We start out with silken, shiny locks and in no time at all, they are yanked off the sides of the face into tight pony tails, a treatment which may well cause receding hair lines in later years. Then we start to backcomb it, as a way of snarling it up and splitting the ends, or we commit minor vandalism with such torture tools as heated tongs, frying dryers and steel combs. Later still, we graduate to serious abuse: risking our health with perming solutions, chemical hair dyes and perhaps the odd application of hydrogen peroxide, a sure method of stripping the last vestiges of shine from the hair.

HAIR POLLUTION

Quite apart from deliberate maltreatment, the hair has a battle on its hands to combat the damaging effects of air pollution, climate and environmental factors. One of the major culprits is the sun: prolonged and repeated exposure dries out the hair and disrupts the cells of the cuticle so that they start to wither and are unable effectively to reflect light. If you continue to roast the hair, it will become dried out, brittle and finally break, and if you have also been using chemical hair dyes or solutions, the sun can really play havoc, distorting the colour and leaving it a kind of orange straw.

Further damage is caused if you don't take the trouble to rinse out salt water or chlorine immediately after swimming, for the sun will drive those harmful minerals and chemicals right into the hair shaft. The effects of such a summer will stay with

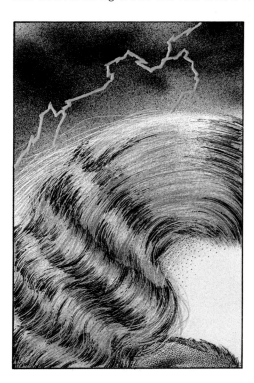

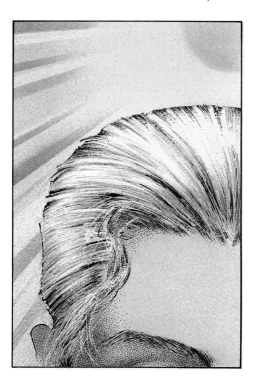

Warning: sprays of pain
If you really must use hair spray, be very careful how you use it. The spray can easily hit the eye of somebody standing behind you, causing great pain, temporary blindness or even severely scratched retinas from plastic particles driven into the eyeballs by the aerosol jet.

D.I.Y: hair protection
Protect the hair with a mixture of one teaspoon each of jojoba, almond and wheatgerm oil; leave the mixture on for 1 hour in the sun. Shampoo the oil out of the hair and apply conditioner as usual.

Hair-raising incidents *are often deliberate: we subject our tresses to shock treatment with crimping and curling tongs (far left) and compound the punishment by baking them in hot sun, drying the strands until they break under the dead weight.*

Treat for limp summer hair
On a lazy summer day, collect flat beer and dilute it with 3 parts water to 1 part beer. Pour it over your hair. The brewery smell with disappear if you give a final rinse with water.

Warning: don a cap
Daily swimming in chlorinated water poses special problems. Algecides interact with chlorine to leave a greenish deposit on blonde hair. Protect your hair with a bathing cap.

you for the next six months because of the damage to the cells that are pushing out new hairs. They will need time to grow long enough for them to be cut off. And by then it is summer again, and the whole process can be repeated!

It does not have to be like that. Before swimming and sunbathing, smear coconut hair gel all over the hair, slicking it back off the face. Every time you come out of the water, rinse the hair and re-apply the gel; use henna wax instead of coconut gel on very dry hair. Alternatively, wear a scarf or hat as protection against the sun; choose a light or white one to deflect the UVA rays. If you have dark hair, you may be lulled into a false sense of security: as you tan so easily, you may think that because your hair does not lighten obviously in the sun, there is no need to worry. On the contrary: dark hair absorbs more UVA rays than fair hair and is therefore damaged more easily.

With sunlamps it is equally important to cover the hair, but avoid conditioner or gel as these can leave nasty burns round the hairline and on the neck. You should also protect the hair when you have a sauna; the temperature can reach 80°C and hair cannot cope at such extreme heat. Wrap towels soaked in cold water round the head and change them as they heat up.

WATER AND WIND DAMAGE

In addition to the havoc caused by chlorinated and salt water, ordinary tap water can be less than beneficial. In hard-water areas particularly, you should always use a hair conditioner to counteract fluoride and other chemicals added to our water supplies. People with greasy hair are often suspicious of conditioners, but the Hair Salad Conditioner conforms to its name, being light, healthy and non-fattening.

Winter poses further hazards to hair. As soon as the central heating comes on and the humidity level drops, the skin and hair are among the first to suffer; furniture, oil paintings and plants are equally damaged by dry air. Unless humidifiers are installed, leave bowls of water in centrally-heated rooms so as to raise the air moisture level; modern heating methods are effective and comfortable, but they also have less desirable side effects, removing moisture from the air and drying out skin and hair, causing premature ageing. You will leave the warm home and go straight out into freezing cold, giving the hair an instant trauma as the temperature plummets to freezing and below. Don't forget a woolly hat or warm scarf; up to 50% of body heat is lost through the head if this is unprotected in subzero temperatures, and your hair will be ruined. Tuck long hair into the coat to protect it against wind and cold, and remove scarf and hat as soon as you return inside to prevent excess production of sweat and oil.

It is easy to protect your hair against temperature catastrophes, and it is common sense to eat a balanced diet to keep your hair – and body – in good condition, but there are situations when you can do little to protect your hair. Serious illness always depletes hair of health and appearance; the body conserves its energies by protecting the major organs, and the hair is the last to receive essential nutrients. Frequently treatment for serious illnesses does actual and severe damage to the hair, notably X-Ray therapy which can cause hair to fall out. Try to treat your hair as gently as possible during illnesses, and avoid harsh petro-chemical shampoos which can speed up hair loss. It is vital for the mental wellbeing of seriously ill people that they are encouraged to maintain their appearance as far as possible; it gives a boost to their confidence and is an essential aid to recovery.

HAIR CARE

HAIR VARIES FROM PERSON TO PERSON AND FROM RACE TO RACE, in colour, length, texture and shape but it can be divided into four basic types of condition: dry, greasy, normal and mixed. Check the Hair Type Chart overleaf to find out the causes for your particular condition so that you can remove some of the external factors. Thereafter refer to the Treatment Chart to find the products that suit your hair. Special attention is given to black Afro hair because the habit of tight braiding and the use of chemical straighteners can both cause black hair to be particularly fragile and dry. It also needs added shine because tight curls cannot absorb light and therefore look dull.

WASHING YOUR HAIR

The purpose of a shampoo is to clean your hair. It is not formulated to protect or repair the hair or to adjust hormonal imbalances such as overactive oil glands. Most shampoos are alkaline in composition because this substance helps to break down

Myth breaker: lather
Lots of lather is not synonymous with a shampoo's effectiveness. Lathering agents are often added to mass-produced shampoos because customers believe, quite wrongly, that more lather means cleaner hair.

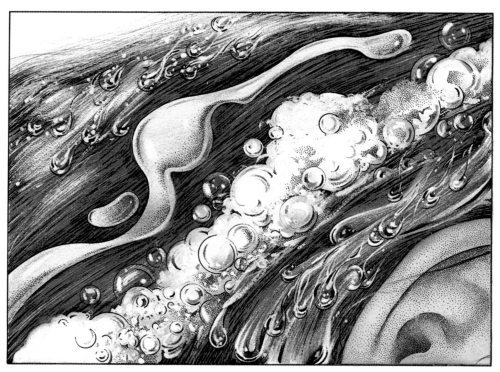

Hair care *starts with more than slapping on the shampoo. Begin with a prewash (bottom) to dislodge oil and grease or to stimulate dry scalps, and follow this with a shampoo suited to the hair type. After thorough rinsing, apply Protein Cream Rinse, Henna Wax or Hair Salad Conditioner, then rinse and rinse again until the hair is completely clean, smooth and silky (top).*

HAIR TYPES

CONDITION	CAUSES	SYMPTOMS	REMEDIES
DRY	Naturally dry hair is usually coarse due to fewer follicles and fewer oil glands. Hair also gets drier with age as the production of sebum slows down. Most dry conditions are due to self-inflicted damage: perms, over-zealous blow drying, and harsh shampoos. Also to insufficient washing and grooming of thick, curly hair because of the effort and pain involved.	Dull, coarse, brittle and easily damaged. Scalp can be tight and flaky. Curly hair is often dry because the bends in the curls open up the hair shafts.	Wash regularly; dry dirty hair is fragile and snarls and splits easily. Before washing, massage the scalp with oil or henna wax to aid circulation and prevent the build-up of dead skin cells which block the hair. Use conditioner at every wash. Avoid heated rollers or dryers, using gel instead and scrunch-dry the hair to protect it and make it shiny.
OILY	Common with fine hair because of more numerous follicles pumping out sebum. Hormonal imbalances, especially in teenagers, also speed up oil production. Poor diet, stress, over-handling and cold weather all contribute to greasy and oily hair.	Lank, dull and stringy; holds style poorly. Unless frequently washed, hair becomes smelly, as it traps sebum, sweat, dirt, dust, tobacco and stale food odours.	Nature remedies this condition, hair becoming drier with age. Until then, wash frequently and as often as you like, shunning petro-chemical and harsh anti-dandruff shampoos. Avoid rich, fatty foods; expose the hair to fresh air for at least 30 min. every day. Use Hair Salad Conditioner as protection on the ends of long hair – shoulder-length hair is about a year old.
NORMAL	Fortunate genetics, healthy diet and sensible precautions.	Glossy throughout; fine hair may be static.	Maintain this happy state of affairs by washing every 3-5 days. Use conditioner to protect the ends; avoid perms. On static hair use Seaweed and Birch Shampoo; the glutinous properties adhere to the hair and give it body.
MIXED	As hair grows long, its condition often changes, the ends becoming dry and brittle. Harmful treatments, sun damage and rough handling exacerbate the mixed condition.	Hair needs frequent washing which seems to make the ends worse.	Alternate a shampoo for greasy hair with one for normal hair, but apply shampoo *only* to the scalp; the rinsing water will carry diluted shampoo through the length of the hair. Use a conditioner as for dry hair, from the ears down *only*. Remove it with diluted lemon or vinegar rinse which will adhere to the unconditioned top of the hair. Then rinse with fresh water.

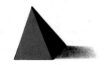

oil and dirt. A few shampoos are labelled as non-alkaline, with a reading below 7.0, the neutral point on the pH scale; often the lather of such shampoos will register as alkaline (above 7.0), and rightly so as otherwise they would not be effective as shampoos. The detergent in Body Shop shampoos is cocomide, derived from coconut, and is a mild but effective cleanser. No petro-chemical bases are used because we believe that such bases progressively penetrate the cuticle and minutely strip off the protective layer.

There is a right way of washing your hair, and a wrong way. Clumsy handling, inadequate rinsing and using too much shampoo are all common mistakes and even professional hairdressers are not always trained to wash and handle hair correctly. Most good salons will let you bring your own shampoo and conditioner, so you can avoid becoming a guinea pig for their latest "miracle" product, as well as saving yourself quite a lot of money.

TEN EASY STEPS TO CLEAN HAIR

1. Treat dry scalps or dry hair to a prewash: massage Jojoba Oil or Aromatherapy Scalp Oil thoroughly into scalp and leave for 20-30 minutes (sitting in a hot bath, the steam will help the oil to penetrate the skin).
2. Never wash your hair while you are taking a bath; the water is dirty, teeming with bits of flaked skin, soap scum and other undesirable elements.
3. Lean over the basin or bath; this position will loosen the skin on the scalp and stimulate blood circulation.
4. Use one capful only of shampoo and spread it between the palms of your hands; for very greasy hair you can dilute the shampoo and repeat the shampooing process. None of our shampoos are heavily diluted.
5. Using the pads of the finger tips, massage the shampoo gently into the scalp. Do not use the length of your hair as a massage pad, and do not massage shampoo into hair growing below chin length.
6. Rinse the hair thoroughly; by the rule of gravity shampoo will travel down the length of your hair, and diluted shampoo is perfect to clean the longer part of the hair which has already had a few hundred shampoos in its lifetime.
7. Rinse again to make sure all traces of shampoo have been removed.
8. Blot dry on a towel. Do not pull or rub the hair as wet hair loses 20% of its natural resilience and elasticity.
9. For long hair use a tablespoon of conditioner, for short hair a teaspoon, and gently fold it into the hair. Do not rub it into the scalp, it is a hair, not a skin, conditioner; use a vulcanized, sawtoothed rubber comb to ease the conditioner through the hair, starting at the root ends.
10. Rinse again and wrap a warm towel round the hair to absorb excess moisture.

DRYING THE HAIR

Whenever possible, let the hair dry naturally of its own accord; blot up excess moisture with a hot towel, but do not wring it out, and avoid using heated appliances. In an emergency, let the hair become almost dry before assaulting it with a hairdryer. Use the lowest temperature setting and never hold the dryer in a fixed position — try blowing it on your hand for a few minutes and see how uncomfortably hot and drying that is; imagine what the same treatment will do for your hair.

Danger: pollution
In Britain, we use 21,000 tonnes of shampoo annually. Consider what happens to it all when it goes down the plug hole. Check that your shampoo is biodegradeable, which means that it will break down in the same way that animals and vegetables decompose and not mess up the fragile ecological balance.

Fact: did you know?
Of all the shampoos sold in Europe, 10% are dandruff shampoos.

HAIR CONDITIONERS

Ironically, conditioners became essential with the advent of effective shampoos after the Second World War. Prior to that, heavy soap shampoos often needed an acid rinse to clear the hair of clogging scum which is why the habit of using vinegar or lemon rinses became popular. Modern shampoos have the ability to clean thoroughly, but at the same time they can leave the hair unmanageable with static. Conditioners are formulated to negate the positive electrical charge that clean hair emits. There is some truth in the advertisers' claim that a conditioner only goes where it is needed, and this is true of all conditioners.

Conditioner makes your hair feel smoother and look shinier and also protects it against the environment and against damage inflicted while grooming. It cuts down on static, reduces fluffiness and smoothes down the cuticles, thus allowing light to reflect evenly from the hair.

Shampoo and conditioner serve different functions, a shampoo opening the pores to clean the hair and a conditioner closing them to protect it. Any scepticism about the benefit of hair conditioners can be dispelled by trying half a head test: use conditioner on one side of the parting only and compare the results.

KITCHEN AND GARDEN REMEDIES

Some practitioners of cosmetic science use just enough natural ingredients in their products to satisfy the Trades Descriptions Act or a passing fancy of fashion. It may be easier and less messy to employ modern synthetics, but natural ingredients have been used for thousands of years in cosmetic tricks and treatments. The exponent of cosmetic science, Ralph Harry, wrote in 1948 "The time is now favourable for research workers to review the usefulness or otherwise of herbal preparations". Unfortunately, this has not materialized on a commercial scale, but there is no reason why you should not try out those natural ingredients which women have used since time immemorial.

Much has been written (and forgotten) about making cosmetic products from kitchen and garden ingredients. When the shampoo and conditioner run out what do you do? You might reach for the soap, or worst still, the washing-up liquid. If you look at those who, with a glint in their eye, brag about washing their hair only in soap, there is always a singular lack of a corresponding glint in their hair — it is inevitably dull and full of scurf, the irremoveable residue left from washing in soap.

Next time you run out of shampoo, try an egg. It is a perfectly effective cleanser and particularly good for dry hair. Separate the yolk from the white. Whisk each separately, then fold them together and massage through dry hair; leave on the head for 5 minutes. Rinse with lukewarm water, never hot, or the egg will scramble.

One of the simplest of herbs is soapwort (*Saponaria officinalis*). It is a perennial garden plant, and it also grows wild as a roadside weed, especially in the West Country. The leaves contain a sap known as saponin, which has been used for centuries to clean the hair. Soapwort was formerly widely used for washing cloth at woollen mills, and it still has a fine reputation among conservationists for cleaning old tapestries and silks; for exactly those qualities of gentle effective cleansing it makes an excellent shampoo. Research in France has proved that soapwort stimulates the sebaceous glands much less than modern shampoo bases and is consequently the solution to greasy and oily hair.

HAIR TREATMENTS AT A GLANCE			
HAIR TYPE	**OCCASIONAL PRECONDITIONER***	**REGULAR SHAMPOO**	**REGULAR CONDITIONER**
DRY			
Fair/fine	Aromatherapy scalp oil	Coconut/Camomile	Protein cream rinse
Fair/thick	Henna wax	Jojoba/Camomile	Henna wax
Dark/fine	Jojoba oil	Henna cream/Rosemary	Protein cream rinse
Dark/thick	Henna wax	Henna cream/Jojoba	Henna wax
GREASY			
Fair/fine	Orange flower water	Camomile powder/ Frequency wash	Hair salad
Fair/thick	—	Camomile powder/Ice blue	Hair salad
Dark/fine	Orange flower water	Frequency wash/Ice blue	Hair salad
Dark/thick	—	Ice blue/Frequency wash	Hair salad
NORMAL			
Fair/fine	Aromatherapy scalp oil	Camomile/Seaweed & birch	Hair salad
Fair/thick	—	Camomile/Jojoba	Protein cream rinse
Dark/fine	Jojoba oil	Rosemary/Orange spice	Hair salad
Dark/thick	Henna wax	Rosemary/Jojoba	Henna wax
MIXED			
Fair/fine	Aromatherapy scalp oil	Camomile/Seaweed & birch	Protein cream rinse
Fair/thick	Aromatherapy scalp oil	Coconut/Camomile	Henna wax
Dark/fine	Orange flower water	Rosemary/Orange spice	Protein cream rinse
Dark/thick	—	Ice blue/Orange spice	Henna wax
BLACK AFRO			
	Jojoba oil	Jojoba/Henna cream	Henna wax
	Use preconditioner once a week, massaging oil or wax into the scalp and leaving it for 30 min. in a steamy atmosphere. Shampoo as usual. Sprinkle orange flower water on to pads of cottonwool and dab along partings made all over the scalp.		

D.I.Y: sun streak spritzers
For fair hair steep 50g of chamomile flowers in 300ml of boiling water, removed from the heat. Leave to cool, then add juice of 1 lemon. Strain and spritz the liquid over the hair when sitting in the sun.

For dark hair add the juice of 1 lemon to 1 cup of strong fresh coffee; strain and cool. Spritz on the hair in the sun.

For aubergine tints use the cooled cooking water from boiled beetroots as a spritzer in the sun. Take care to keep it off clothes or it will stain.

Natural cleansers: *a beaten egg shampoo for dry hair. Lemon juice for greasy hair, as a rinse or a conditioner, or with a chamomile infusion as a spritzer on fine hair (far right).*

Another plant rich in saponin is the so-called soap bark tree, *Quillaia saponaria;* the compound is obtained from the powdered bark, but as the tree is native to South America, you will have to obtain the powder from a herbalist, or a joke shop. If you sniff it you will be sneezing so badly that shampooing is out of the question, which is why the powder is most commonly used for sneezing powders.

Kitchen cupboard staples for hair care include lemon and vinegar which have been used generation after generation as pH-balanced hair conditioners. They were essential with soap-based shampoos to lift off the alkaline scum, and they still do an effective job on greasy hair by closing the cuticles and leaving the hair shiny. Use a weak solution of either as a final rinse.

Elderberries have been a cosmetic aid for centuries. The Romans used them to dye their hair, but in our experiments we have found them to be fairly useless for this purpose. What they do really well is condition the hair. The natural acids and pectins in elderberries make the hair shiny and manageable. For a prewash conditioner, crush fresh elderberries, strain the juice and dilute it with an equal amount of water. Pour through the hair 5 minutes before washing, then rinse out. The distinctive smell will not linger and should not put you off one of the best natural conditioners.

You can boost the level of natural ingredients in your shampoo or conditioner by adding infusions as supplements. Chamomile will brighten and add shine to blonde hair; henna gives shine and body to dark hair, and rosemary has the added bonus of saponin with its cleansing properties. To make an infusion steep 25g of herbs in

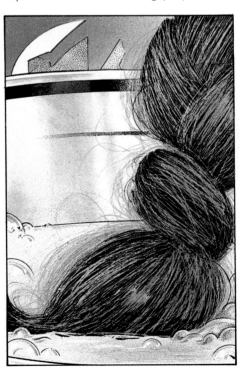

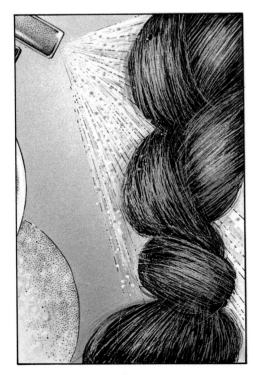

300ml of boiling water for 30 minutes, then strain. You can dilute a shampoo with 50% of the infusion, and a conditioner with 25%.

Mint is another, readily available plant useful in hair care. An excellent scalp treatment can be made by soaking garden mint in almond oil: steep 50g mint leaves in 225ml almond oil for two weeks, then strain it through muslin. Discard the mint and repeat the process, using the original almond oil and another 50g of fresh mint leaves. Strain the oil after a couple of weeks and keep it in a stoppered bottle. Massage the oil regularly into the scalp; it will help to slow down hair fall due to the anti-oxidant effect of the menthol in the mint. If you substitute rosemary for mint you have an effective massage oil against dandruff.

One of the best natural ingredients comes from the green colouring matter in plants, chlorophyll. Nettles, for example, contain nearly 1% chlorophyll, in addition to several curative minerals, including iron; herbalists have been using nettles for sore scalps ever since the Romans introduced the plant. We also use Persian sedra in Camomile Powder Shampoo because it cleans the hair by absorbing dirt and grease, and is easily rinsed out; it is particularly effective for greasy hair and for giving body. Soil itself has many excellent properties, and some clays will clean the hair as well as any modern shampoo. One favourite is Moroccan mud, known as rhassoul mud, which is mined from the Atlas Mountains. You can buy it dried, and mixed with water and used as a shampoo it makes an effective cleanser for greasy hair and an excellent dandruff treatment; an additional bonus from both sedra and rhassoul is

Hint: scalp cleansing
Long hair, which for one reason or another cannot be washed frequently, becomes clean and fresh-smelling if a lime, cut into thin slices is rubbed thoroughly over the scalp.

Beauty hint: quick lifts
If you have neither energy nor time to wash your hair, use orris root as a dry shampoo. Brush 25g of orris root through the hair to remove grease and make the hair smell fresh. Make sure that you brush out all traces of the powder.

Body builders *are present in everyday ingredients like beer (far left); use it diluted as a final rinse on limp hair. Egg yolks are rich in protein and, mixed with diluted shampoo, ideal for greasy hair; follow with a rinse or spritzer of chamomile infusion.*

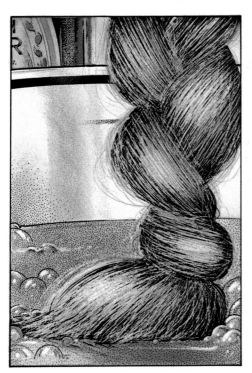
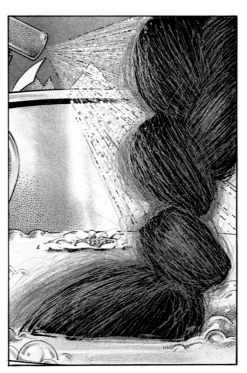

Overleaf *"No other part of the body has such incredible flexibility. Hair is fascinating stuff, a glorious material to play with and enjoy."*

that you end up with incredibly soft hands. If you have difficulty obtaining rhassoul, Fuller's Earth and kaolin make good substitutes. Mix them to a paste with water and apply as a mud pack to the hair. Leave it on for 10 minutes before rinsing it out.

BLACK AFRO HAIR
Only in recent years has the care of black hair been given any attention in Europe and it is still difficult to get good advice outside large cities. Afro hair is essentially different because the shape of each hair is elliptical rather than round. One fascinating result of this difference is that a black person cannot catch head lice from a white person! The vermin that infest Caucasian hair have claws designed to grip round hair shafts; they are impotent on elliptical hair shafts and *vice versa*.

Black hair is an effective block to the damaging effects of UVA sun rays. The structure of each curl ensures that rays are picked up at several angles and absorbed into the hair, thereby protecting the head and keeping it cool. However, the same structure means that the hair is often very dry as the curls allow moisture to escape from the hair shaft, and it becomes difficult for sebum to travel down and lubricate the hair. It also makes the hair more brittle as the curls loop into each other and get tangled; the tight bends of the curls cause the cuticles to open out and fray. It is often thought that black hair grows slower than other racial hair types, but evidence suggests that it simply breaks off more easily and is damaged by chemical treatments, such as straighteners.

Although black Afro hair is invariably dry, it does not necessarily follow that the scalp is also dry. The scalp is skin and if face and body skin are dry, the scalp will be equally so. The most common mistake is to apply lots of oils to dry hair on a greasy scalp, which only serves to block the follicles. Treat such greasy skin before washing by separating the hair into sections and dabbing with cottonwool soaked in orange flower water along the partings. This will lift excess oil and tone the skin. Shampoo gently, kneading the scalp as you wash the hair. Use shampoo sparingly and leave it on the hair for a few minutes. Apply conditioner to the hair, *not to the scalp*.

For dry skin, massage oil well into the scalp for 5-10 minutes, then gently shampoo it out and apply conditioner. You can use a light hair dressing such as Macassar oil to prevent the scalp and hair from drying out.

INGROWING HAIR
Black hair is coarse and forms such tight curls that it can start to grow into the skin. When this happens, the skin becomes inflamed and the follicles can be damaged, leading to hair loss. It is more noticeable on men's facial hair as shaving aggravates the problem by keeping the hair very short. If the problem persists, it is worth considering a beard. Ingrowing hair becomes more serious if it has been treated with chemical straighteners or hair dyes. The introduction of these chemicals into the skin can affect the general health, and the risks associated with hair dyes are obviously more serious in this context.

HAIR STRAIGHTENERS
Only the stronger of these chemical compounds work well on black hair; some are made of sodium hydroxides which weaken the hair substantially so that it becomes brittle and easily breaks off. Trichologists report that the use of these products is the

JOJOBA

Many cosmetic products used to be based on the oil extracted from the blubber of the sperm whale.

When the sperm whale became an endangered species in 1970, research for an alternative centred on jojoba.

Jojoba thrives in arid desert regions, tolerating strong winds, fierce heat and prolonged drought.

Jojoba oil closely resembles sperm whale oil in composition containing a wax-like substance suspended in alcohol.

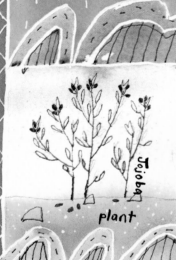

Jojoba plant

Jojoba is suitable for the treatment of pimples and acne.

For centuries Jojoba was valued only by the Mohave and Apache Indian tribes for shining their hair.

Jojoba is totally pure and the oil is light, non-greasy and readily absorbed by the skin.

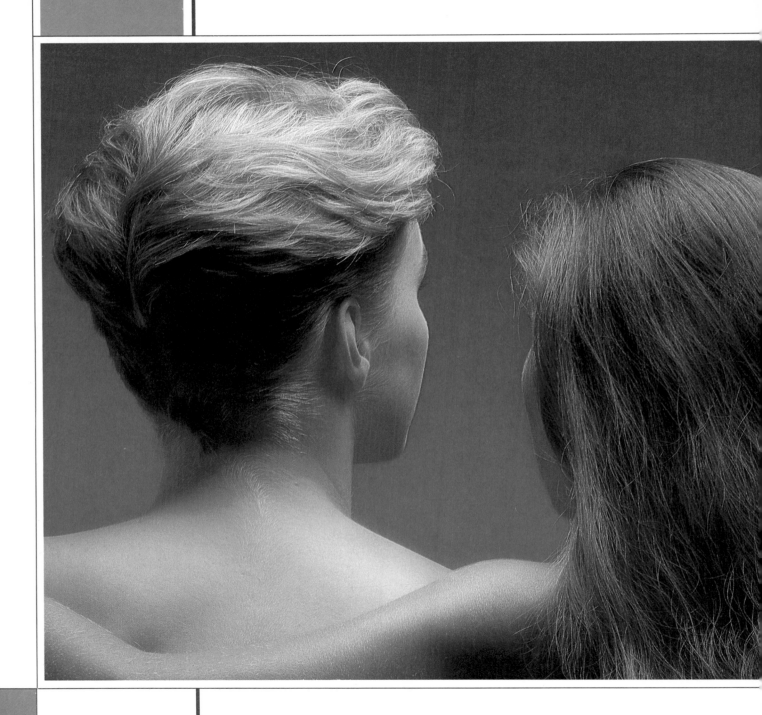

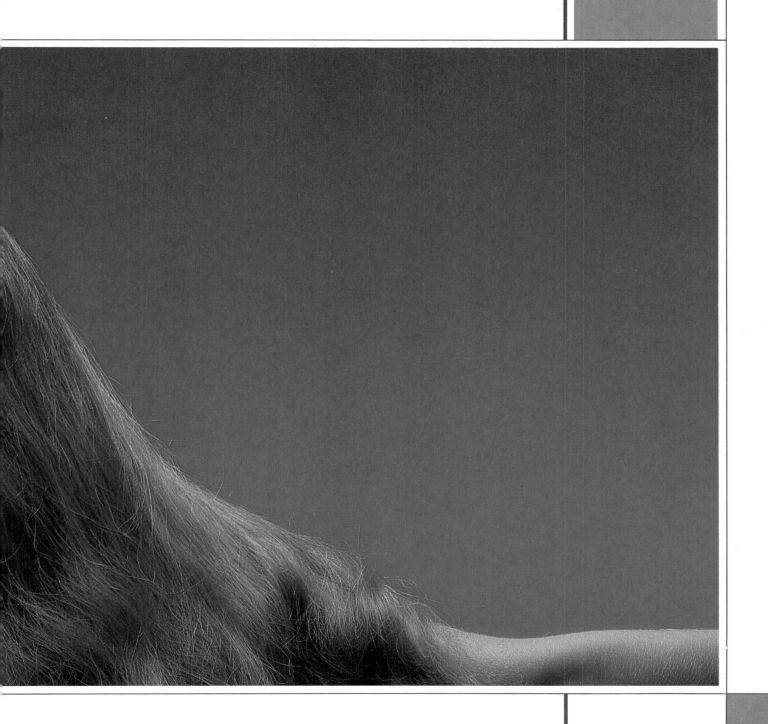

HENNA

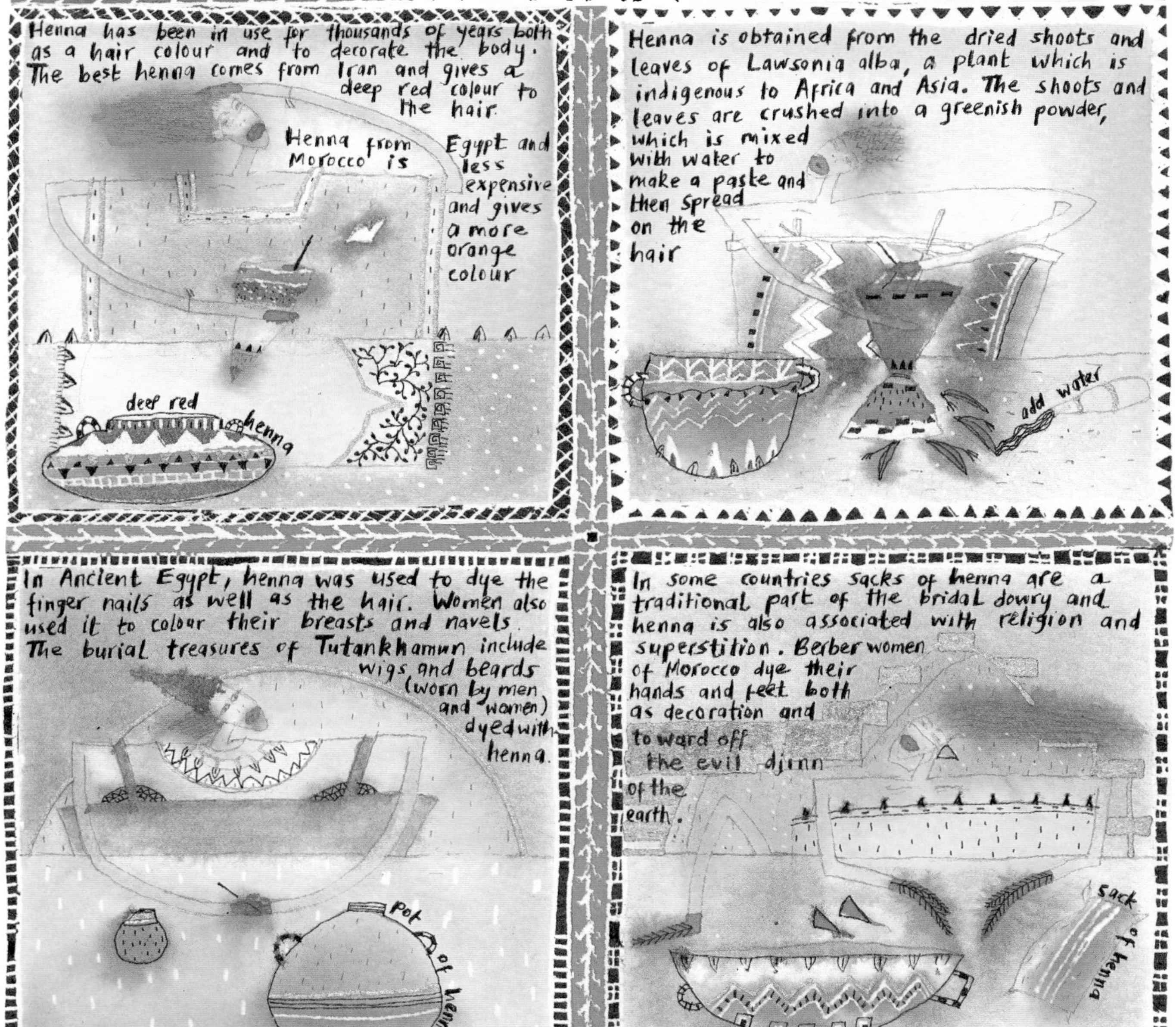

Henna has been in use for thousands of years both as a hair colour and to decorate the body. The best henna comes from Iran and gives a deep red colour to the hair.

Henna from Morocco is Egypt and less expensive and gives a more orange colour

Henna is obtained from the dried shoots and leaves of Lawsonia alba, a plant which is indigenous to Africa and Asia. The shoots and leaves are crushed into a greenish powder, which is mixed with water to make a paste and then spread on the hair

deep red henna

add water

In Ancient Egypt, henna was used to dye the finger nails as well as the hair. Women also used it to colour their breasts and navels. The burial treasures of Tutankhamun include wigs and beards (worn by men and women) dyed with henna.

pot of henna

In some countries sacks of henna are a traditional part of the bridal dowry and henna is also associated with religion and superstition. Berber women of Morocco dye their hands and feet both as decoration and to ward off the evil djinn of the earth.

sack of henna

most common cause of hair loss amongst black people. For the odd occasion hot brushing will straighten the hair to some extent without causing the damage that chemical straighteners wreak, or you can try the turban method: section the hair in the middle and create a turban effect by wrapping the front of one section across the head over a large roller; bring the front of the other side across, and alternate the hair wraps until the whole head has been covered. This method is not suitable on damp and humid days as the hair absorbs moisture and will quickly revert to curls.

BRAIDING

The sculptural look of rows of corn and tight plaits is attractive, but should not be used all the time. The constant strain of pulling the hair into tight braids can cause hair loss, particularly around the hair line. Braided hair is very easy to wash: use a shower attachment and run the water along the partings so that the shampoo washes through the braids. You can also cover the hair with a nylon stocking to keep the braids neatly in place and wash through the stocking. Braids can be left for a few weeks as they gradually loosen as the hair grows.

Steaming is possibly the best method for preventing hair breakage and for making the hair feel soft. Massage Henna Wax well into the hair and cover with hot towels or with a plastic cap. Sit in a hot steamy bath or use a steaming appliance on the hair for 15 minutes. Shampoo the oil out of the hair and afterwards condition as usual.

SCALP MASSAGE

Unlike other massages, scalp massage does not involve stripping and an inferiority complex about looking like a lump of lard. A massage medium is not really necessary either as the scalp's own oils will provide enough lubrication to do a good job. However, you do need a partner; massaging your own scalp is ineffective – the minute you raise your arms, the interacting muscles pull tight, and you will end up with the feeling that the scalp is cemented to the skull. Added to this, the blood drains from your arms and they go numb before they have begun to do any good.

Along with foot massage (reflexology), having your scalp massaged is one of the nicest and most relaxing sensations and ideal for easing tension. In addition, scalp massage encourages any oils used to penetrate the skin; the therapeutic qualities of aromatherapy oils in particular help to increase the blood supply to the surface of the skin. This in turn encourages all the working parts, such as hair growth, shedding of dead skin, etc., to function normally. Scalp massage tones the hair as well as the scalp muscles and improves the manageability of the hair.

Have the "victim", a towel round her shoulders, sitting in a comfortable armchair or on cushions at your feet, supported by your legs. Discourage smoking which will get up your nose and irritate you, reading which entails a forward position inappropriate for massage, and crossing of the legs which restricts blood circulation.

Apply a little scalp or almond oil with cottonwool to the scalp and divide the hair into partings about 3cm apart. Start at the nape of the neck and work towards the front of the head, using only the balls of your fingers to exert gentle pressure, and knead the scalp. You should be able to feel it move while the head stays still. Avoid the sensitive areas at the temples and behind the ears. Concentrate on the top and back of the head, interlacing the fingers as you cross the top.

D.I.Y: scalp massage
Cup your hands so that contact with scalp comes from the finger pads and the base of the palms. Make circular movements of the scalp over a small area for 1 minute before moving to an adjacent area. Continue until the whole scalp has been covered.

HAIR PROBLEMS

Bonus
One advantage of growing old is that you won't get dandruff; it simply disappears after the late 60s.

Opposite: *dry hair problems can stem from naturally dry skin, sloppy rinsing or flaking sunburn. Use a conditioner after every wash; don't scrunch it in but comb it through the clean hair, from the roots to the tips, to leave the hair smooth and shiny.*

A NORMAL SCALP HAS BETWEEN 24 AND 40 LAYERS OF DEAD CELLS which are constantly moving up to the surface where they are shed. The cycle for each layer takes 28 days. Although we tend to describe flaking scalps as dandruff, true dandruff is skin cells flaking 20-30 layers deep, thus exposing the cells before they have hardened and are ready to be shed. This is why dandruff is often associated with an irritated scalp. Just as nails torn to the quick are inflamed and painful, scalp cells which have not hardened and are not ready to be shed make the skin feel tender and itchy.

There are as many theories regarding the causes of dandruff as there are about its nature. The strongest evidence suggests it is a bacterial infection, coupled with accelerated hormonal reaction which pushes out new skin cells without giving the old cells a chance to be shed. It is almost universally agreed that dandruff is stress-related; scalp massage is particularly helpful as it has the dual function of aiding circulation and at the same time relieving tension and easing headaches and constriction of the scalp.

DANDRUFF

If you have dry skin on your face and body, you can expect the scalp to be dry too. This can be easily remedied by massaging Jojoba Oil into the scalp 10 minutes before washing your hair. The massage will aid circulation, and the oil will keep the skin lubricated and protected without leaving it greasy, as any excess will be shampooed out. Brutally scouring the scalp as you brush your hair is not helpful. Choose a brush without scratchy pointed ends; it can be rubber, nylon or bristle but the ends must be rounded. Some mothers brush their childrens' hair as if they were getting a grappling iron into a cliff face. This is counter-productive. It will damage the hair and the scalp, the children will soon rebel and refuse ever to brush their hair at all, and family harmony will suffer.

What is described as a flaking scalp is often the residue of shampoo which has not been thoroughly rinsed out. In areas where the water is hard, always use conditioner on your hair to get rid of any mineral traces in the water. As a general rule always rinse the hair twice as much as you think necessary.

Don't forget your scalp can get sunburnt. Too much exposure to the sun will cause the skin to peel in exactly the same way as it peels on the rest of your body. Protect hair and scalp with a hat.

If you have an oily complexion, your scalp will probably also be greasy. The flaking cells associated with greasy hair are usually caused by the follicles getting blocked and skin cells sticking to the sebum. Before washing your hair, make partings all over the scalp and dab it with cottonwool soaked in orange flower water to absorb excess sebum and lift off the skin cells. You can try the same remedy between washes if you notice scales building up.

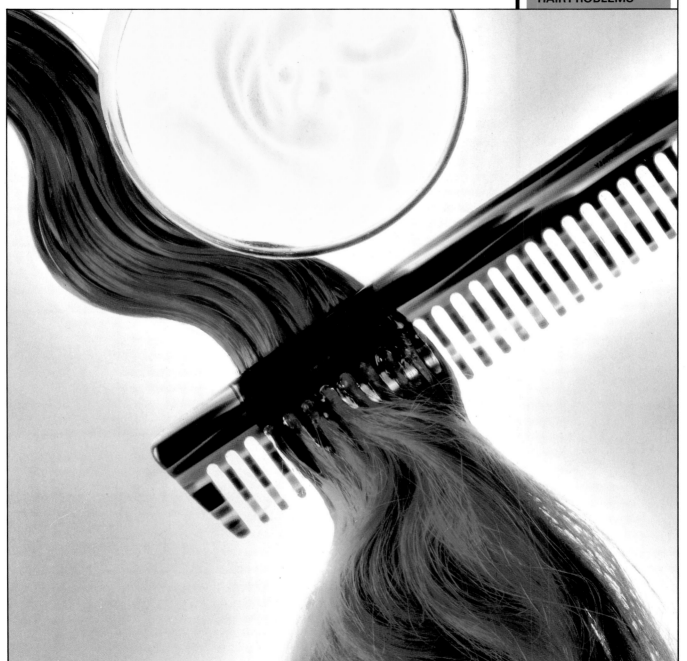

Babies are often born with cradle cap, a crust on their scalps, usually over the "soft spot". Mothers are rightly concerned about touching this vulnerable area and often leave the cradle cap alone. The crust is formed of natural secretions and will disappear quickly if treated with care: heat a little almond oil to lukewarm and apply it very gently to the scalp with cottonwool. Do not rub or push at the scalp in any way. Wash the baby's head with Goat's Milk Soap, first dampening the scalp with a wet sponge, then massaging it gently with the *palms* of your hands.

Many of the anti-dandruff shampoos on the market are harsh in themselves. One common ingredient in these products is zinc pyrithione which tends to make the hair look dull and should not be used regularly. Selenium sulphide, another common ingredient, has caused concern among experts in the heavy-metal poison field. It is a highly toxic anti-bacterial agent which can be absorbed through the skin. Continued use of products containing this substance may cause a harmful build up of levels of minerals which can lead to premature ageing.

If none of these conditions apply, a flaking or itching scalp may be caused by any of the following:

COMMON DANDRUFF Skin flakes fall off easily. They may be grey-white or yellowish in colour and are worst over the ears, dropping on to the shoulders. The scalp usually feels itchy.

NEURODERMATITIS The base of the scalp will be very itchy and when you scratch it, more scales appear. This condition is often associated with the menopause.

PITYRIASIS Scales build up along the shafts of the hair. If left unattended the condition can lead to hair loss.

PSORIASIS This disease can affect the whole body with loose silver-white scales; the skin beneath will be red and itchy. It is often chronic, and difficult to cure; sunlight would appear to ease the condition which requires medical attention.

If you suspect the flaking condition of your scalp to be other than common dandruff or cannot identify the cause of the condition, consult your doctor or a qualified trichologist.

DANDRUFF AND FLAKING SCALP TREATMENT			
	PREWASH	WASH	CONDITIONER
DANDRUFF	AROMATHERAPY SCALP OIL	ORANGE SPICE SHAMPOO	PROTEIN CREAM RINSE
DRY HAIR/ DRY SCALP	JOJOBA OIL	JOJOBA OR ORANGE SPICE SHAMPOO	HENNA WAX
GREASY HAIR/ FLAKING SCALP	ORANGE FLOWER WATER	ICE BLUE SHAMPOO OR ORANGE SPICE SHAMPOO	HAIR SALAD CONDITIONER

It is essential to use a prewash treatment as this lifts the dead skin cells that have built up. The accompanying gentle massage will stimulate circulation and allow the shampoo to work effectively.

HAIR TREATMENT PRODUCTS

The Body Shop produced the first medicated shampoo in which the medication comes entirely from the properties of herb and spice oils: *Orange Spice Shampoo* contains infusions of nettle and rosemary to cleanse and stimulate the scalp, a blend of anti-microbial essential oils to keep the scalp free of infection, and essential oil of cinnamon leaf, clove, thyme and vetivert (cuscus root), to penetrate the scalp and prevent the cells from clumping together.

Aromatherapy Scalp Oil is a blend of aromatic oils, including lavender oil to stimulate the blood vessels feeding the follicles, juniper oil to strengthen skin and scalp tissues, cypress oil to lubricate and soothe the scalp, rosemary oil, a known antiseptic, to increase hair growth, wheatgerm oil, an anti-oxidant, to help slow down hair loss, and almond oil to cleanse the scalp and remove the scales.

HAIR LOSS

Hair loss has always induced panic: "A person, phlegmatic to the point of accepting with utmost serenity the loss of property or money, does not fail to become dejected and panicky at the sight of his first combful of fallen hairs. A battleship more or less is of relatively little importance to him when he sees a vision of himself denuded of his hair, his scalp a skating rink for venturesome flies". This sorry view of male baldness comes from the 1930s when you might think there were more pressing worries to hand. Men's virility and women's femininity are inextricably bound up with the hairs on their heads. Trichologists report a high increase every autumn in clients panicking that they might be going bald. It is usually due to the seasonal pattern of hair loss with the autumn as the "fall" period. For hair to be seen as thinning you need to lose between 40-50% from one area. Noticeable hair loss means that too much of the hair is in the Catogen Phase at one time, and it is important to establish why.

WHAT CAUSES HAIR LOSS?

During pregnancy hair is usually at its best and appears thicker than usual. This is because you retain the hairs that you would normally lose over the nine months. With the sudden hormonal dip at childbirth you start to lose the extra hairs you have stored as well as the ones you would lose anyway. A supplement of brewers' yeast tablets will help to restore the hair.

You may experience hair loss if you have been on a strict diet which does not cover all the bodily needs for essential nutrients. The body, believing itself to be starving, will conserve essential nutrients for the major organs before supplying hair and nails. For that reason hair and nails act as efficient early warning systems to your health. The remedy is simple: eat a balanced diet and avoid diet fads.

Severe stress can cause temporary hair loss. It has been noted that the occurrence of hair loss is on the increase among some women who have high-stress jobs, mimicking the increase in other stress-induced diseases previously associated with men. It is possible that such women produce a high quantity of the male hormone, testosterone. It will be interesting to note over coming decades if the incidence of

Warning: think about it! Keep chemical anti-dandruff shampoos out of the reach of children. The probable lethal dose if swallowed by a child is less than 25ml.

Myth breaker: rub-a-dub The only magic of hair restoring potions, from Hippocrates to the present, probably comes from all the rubbing in!

41

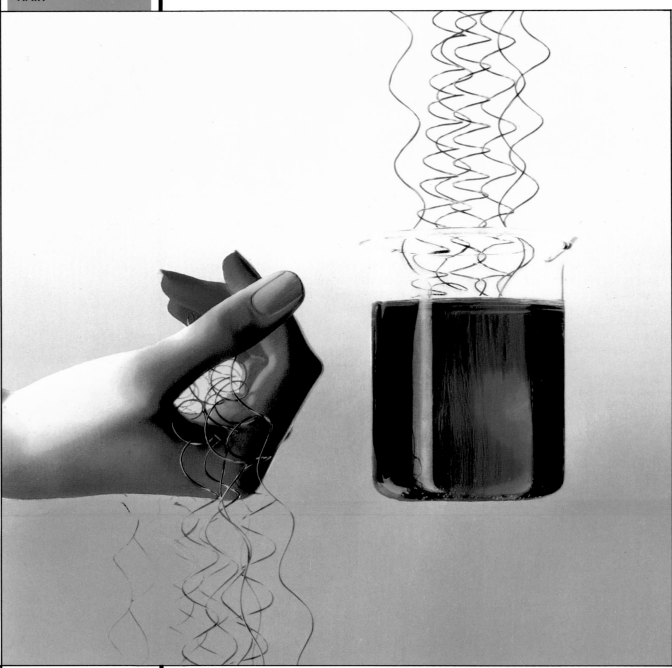

the genetic male-pattern baldness also occurs in women. As with all stress-induced symptoms, relaxation techniques do help and regular scalp massages can minimize the effects of stress.

The menopause is most commonly accompanied by hair loss, particularly in women who have a quick menopause. Hormone treatments administered to alleviate other menopausal problems can minimize hair loss, but it is generally inevitable that some hair thinning will take place in women between the ages of 45-55. This could be the time to reconsider your hair style and perhaps change to a shorter cut to make the hair look thicker.

Male-pattern baldness cannot happen before puberty. The hormonal activity which triggers puberty also triggers off this genetic pattern, said to be inherited through the female line. Typically the greatest hair loss occurs at the front and central regions of the scalp. Hair follicles which have been genetically programmed to cease producing hair will eventually stop functioning. The use of female hormones to counteract this is not advisable because of other unwanted female characteristics. There is no known cure for the condition, and hair transplants are still a risky and expensive undertaking. However, you can slow down the balding process by avoiding harsh chemical treatments.

Recent research in Sweden would appear to indicate benefits from anti-oxidants to slow down hair loss. We have used this research to formulate Ice Blue Shampoo in which menthol, a natural anti-oxidant, is combined with peppermint oil to encourage a good blood supply to the scalp. The importance of massage cannot be overstated, and the shampoo should be kneaded gently into the scalp or used in conjunction with Aromatherapy Scalp Oil to stimulate circulation.

Trichotillomania is the scientific term for hair pulling, a form of self-abuse most commonly found in adolescent girls. It may start as a nervous habit, twisting and tugging at the hair, and result in unsightly bald patches. Professional advice should be sought early as continuous hair pulling can damage the follicles and cause regrowth to be kinked.

HAIR LICE

A major comeback of head lice was reported in the mid-1970s by the London School of Hygiene and Tropical Medicine when 200,000 school children were found to be infested. Contrary to popular belief, **lice love clean short hair** and are no respecters of class or income bracket. Preparations available from chemists are effective; they should be used as treatment, not as preventive measures because the chemical properties will damage the condition of the hair with frequent use. Sufferers often continue using them because they can still see little white sacs adhering to the hairs. If the preparations have been used correctly, the sacs will be dead. They cement themselves to the hair with a gluey substance; the best way of getting rid of them is to use a vinegar solution to dissolve the glue and a fine-toothed comb to extract the sacs from the hair.

SUPERFLUOUS HAIR

Historically, body hair has had a chequered past: the ancient Greeks and Romans removed all trace of body hair, including pubic hair, but generally art provides few clues to the changing attitudes to female body hair. Painters like Cézanne included it

Fact: did you know?
Barbers formerly acted as medicine men, and the traditional barber's pole was in fact the pole used for blood letting. The white stripes symbolize the bandages which were kept ready tied to the pole. The small bowl beneath was used for shaving, not for catching the blood!

Fact: of lice
Fashionable ladies of earlier centuries commonly wore a small container of antiseptic fluid in the cleavage. As lice fell from the hair, they splashed to their death in the liquid.

Opposite: *a lock of hair has the same bounce and resilience as strands of fine copper wire, but when it is wet, it loses part of its strength because it stretches by more than half its length.*

43

Fact: the kiss of death
Depilation was important to third-century Romans; they used a depilatory cream based on yellow arsenic which would reduce the hair to a soft mess. The chief — and fatal — disadvantage came from kissing or inadvertently licking the hands.

Warning: throw-out
Banish these items:
Heated rollers
Hair spray
Metal combs
Plain rubber bands
Scratchy brushes

Rubber bands *are anathema to hair, strangling it and damaging the cortex layer from which its strength and elasticity come. Plain rubber bands (top) disintegrate and snap; throw them out and use fabric-covered bands instead.*

in his nude studies while Matisse, 30 years Cézanne's junior, omitted it. Ruskin's ignorance of the female form in any guise other than that of classical statues contributed to his inability to consummate his marriage. His wife, Effie Gray, wrote, "He told me his true reason . . . that he had imagined women were quite different to what he saw I was, and the reason he did not make me his wife was that he was quite disgusted with my person the first evening". Nor are such preferences confined to the West. In Uganda, it is common practice for all body hair to be removed by applying a special liquid resin to their skin, leaving it to harden and then ripping off the dry resin and hairs in one painful operation.

Females have as much potential to be hairy as men; they have as many hair follicles as men, but most of these usually remain dormant. Hormonal changes at the menopause can result in the development of coarser body hair which is generally seen as undesirable. Oestrogen pills sometimes prescribed for difficult menopauses can restrict the growth of unwanted hair.

DEPILATORY METHODS

In the 1960s and 70s a more natural approach to body hair was predicted, and a national Sunday newspaper proclaimed that "by 1975 every pretty girl will have hairy legs otherwise she will look old-fashioned". These halcyon days have failed to materialize and the problem is still how to remove unwanted hair. Several methods are recommended, some more efficient than others, and none of them painless.

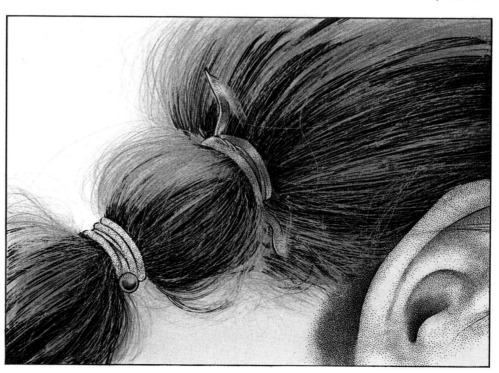

Shaving.

Unless you use an electric razor, use shaving cream or soap to soften the hair and prevent the razor from snagging the skin. Always shave in the direction of hair growth to prevent hair from growing in. If you cut yourself while shaving in the bath, get out quickly as hot water increases the blood flow; when the bleeding stops, smear the area with Wheatgerm Oil to prevent scarring.

Pros and cons Shaving is quick, cheap and efficient; it does not increase hair growth but the skin will feel stubbly. *Never* shave on your face, the bikini line or around the nipples.

Pumice Stone

This is the oldest of all remedies. Scrub with the stone over small skin areas at a time. It is best used as a follow-up to other methods.

Pros and cons Ineffective on long coarse hair and just as painful as other methods.

Tweezing/Plucking

Numb the area with an ice cube and pluck out one hair at a time.

Pros and cons Plucking can stimulate hair growth, so pluck eyebrows only and never pluck hair out of a mole.

Waxing

Melt the wax over gentle heat and leave it to cool to a bearable temperature. For the legs it is easiest to apply the wax to strips of gauze cut to the length from knee to ankle; lightly dusting the legs with talcum powder, smooth down the gauze strips in the direction of hair growth and rip them up from the ankles to the knees.

Pros and cons Regrowth is slow and finer. Do not wax sensitive or sunburnt skin. Use cold wax strips for face and nipples.

Electrolysis

It is a slow process and can cause local discomfort, but for anyone who is distressed over superfluous hair electrolysis offers a permanent if expensive solution. If the skin registers any sign of damage or inflammation within 24 hours after treatment cancel your next appointment. **Do not try home electrolysis kits;** scarring can result if the needle is wrongly inserted.

Myth breaker: stubbly chins
Shaving does not make hair grow coarse and bristly – it just feels that way because shaving cuts off the tapered ends of the hairs.

HAIR COLOUR

HAIR COLOUR IS ONE OF THE FEW PHYSICAL ATTRIBUTES THAT WE do not have to learn to live with. Most features cannot be altered, but if you dislike the colour of your hair, you can change it. It is quick, dramatic, painless, cheap and, given a little time, reversible. You may decide you cannot live with the new colour, but that too can be changed.

People have been dyeing their hair for thousands of years with all manner of strange substances: ash, wine, blood, roots and flowers were all commonly tried as hair dyes. Pliny recorded a particularly unpleasant recipe for dyeing white hair, which included leeches and vinegar fermenting in a lead vessel with the odd earthworm thrown in for good measure. He added a cautionary note that oil should be held in the mouth while applying the dye to prevent the teeth from going black.

The first chemical hair dye was patented by Monnet et Cie in Paris in 1883. It was based on an aniline dye called paraphenylenediamine, which was used in the dyeing of textiles. It seemed a logical progression to try out this particular dye on the hair as

Tip: keeping grey hair at bay
1. Eat a balanced diet.
2. Eat yoghourt regularly.
3. Give up smoking.
4. Dr Seive of Cornell University claims to have changed the colour of 300 of his patients from grey to their natural colour by giving them 50mg of PABA daily. The Body Shop does not endorse the practice of taking PABA internally.
5. Try a D.I.Y. colour rinse, herbal not chemical.

Danger: pregnancy
Don't use chemical hair
dyes when you are
pregnant. The chemicals
can enter the body and
damage the foetus.

Warning: don't do it!
Never use chemical hair
dyes on eyelashes,
eyebrows or any other
body hair.

Danger: pains for beauty
Permanent hair dyes are
more likely to cause allergic
reactions than any other
cosmetic preparations. The
symptoms can be
terrifying: the head may
swell as large as a football,
and swelling of the tongue
can cause asphyxiation.
*Permanent hair dyes
should be patch-tested 24
hours before use*

Opposite: *chemical
laboratory experiments are
conducted in the sterile
atmosphere of an operating
theatre, yet consumers are
encouraged to expose their
hair and skin to potentially
lethal preparations.*

women had traditionally used vegetable textile dyes, such as beetroot juice, saffron and turmeric, on their hair. That first experiment began the upsurge in the use of chemical dyes which became prevalent in the early 20th century, at the expense of vegetable dyes. The immediate success and attraction of such hair dyes are easily understood: they could instantly and miraculously colour a full head of white hair and transform other hair colours.

HOW CHEMICAL HAIR DYES WORK

Permanent hair colours are aniline dyes. They must stay on the head for some time in order to oxidize slowly so as to give the desired colour. The pigment lodges in the cortex and changes the structure of the hair. Initially, as the colour is seen through the compact cortex, the hair looks shiny and healthy. However, repeated applications swell the cortex and damage the cuticles, and the hair begins to look dull and lifeless. Because the colour is permanent and regrowth can be very noticeable, repeat applications must be made, with the result that the hair may end up badly damaged and brittle.

Temporary and semi-permanent colour rinses coat the hair. They can change the colour by a couple of shades, but if a great change is required they can appear patchy and uneven. By far the most important aspect of chemical hair dyes is not the damage done to the hair – after all, hair can be cut off and will grow out again. The really important thing to consider before you contemplate a chemical hair dye is the possible risk to your health.

HAIR DYES AND CANCER?

In Britain alone, one woman in five dyes her hair, and any health risk associated with hair dyes must be taken very seriously. As early as 1938, cosmetic legislation was prompted in the US by blinding and death caused by coal tar-based hair dyes. By powerful lobbying, manufacturers and promoters of these products managed to exempt hair dyes from the very Food, Drug and Cosmetic Act designed to control them. The Act merely required manufacturers to include a warning notice stating "CAUTION – this product contains ingredients which may cause skin irritations on certain individuals, and a preliminary test according to the accompanying instructions should be made first. This product must not be used for dyeing eyelashes or eyebrows: to do so may cause blindness".

In 1970, tests were conducted in America to determine the effects of 2,4-TDA, a fixative mainly used in dark shades of permanent and semi-permanent hair dyes. The tests sought to explain why women using two kinds of commonly available hair dyes complained of passing black urine. *As no explanation could be found the products continued to be on sale without alteration.*

In 1975 Dr Bruce Ames conducted a series of tests on common commercial products to detect which, if any, might be cancer-inducing. Two common products, cigarette tar smoke and a permanent hair dye, showed as mutagens. Further tests revealed that 89% of chemical hair dyes could cause mutation. As all carcinogens are mutagens, these conclusions suggested that the products should be further investigated. Following the 1970 tests which had highlighted the side effects of 2,4-TDA, manufacturers had begun to replace this with 2,4-DAA. Dr Ames found this substance to be 30 times MORE active as a mutagen.

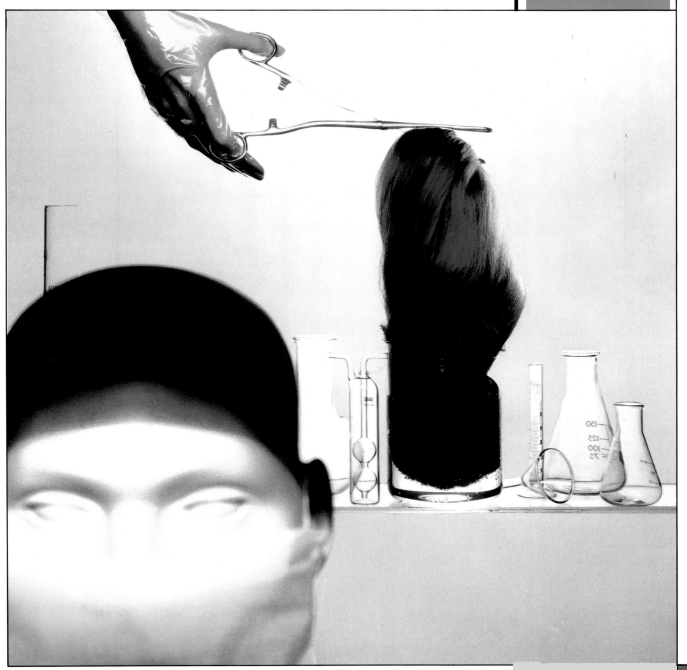

USING HERBAL HAIR COLOURS

NATURAL HAIR COLOUR	BLONDE HERBAL HAIR COLOUR	EGYPTIAN HENNA	EXTRA RED HERBAL HAIR COLOUR	RICH RED BROWN HERBAL HAIR COLOUR	DARK BROWN HERBAL HAIR COLOUR	CHAMOMILE FLOWERS
BLACK	X	2-6 hours red lights	2-6 hours red lights	2-6 hours red lights	2-6 hours deep shine	X
DARK BROWN	X	2-4 hours red lights	1-4 hours auburn	1-4 hours chestnut	1-6 hours walnut	X
MID BROWN	1-2 hours highlights	1-3 hours auburn	1-3 hours auburn	1-4 hours chestnut	1-4 hours dark brown	rinse highlights
LIGHT BROWN	1-2 hours golden lights	½-1 hour red	½-1 hour gold/red	½-1 hour auburn	½-2 hours dark brown	rinse gold lights
DARK BLONDE	½-1 hour gold/blonde	¼-½ hour ginger	X	X	X	rinse lightens
WHITE BLONDE	X	X	X	X	X	rinse brightens
REDHEADS	¼-1 hour blonde lights	¼-1 hour ginger	¼-1 hour red	¼-1 hour auburn	¼-1 hour chestnut	rinse lightens
WHITE	¼-½ hour golden/blonde	X	X	X	X	rinse brightens

Further damaging evidence came from a survey in California of 3000 female cancer deaths which suggests that beauticians in regular contact with chemical hair dyes appear to have a ten times greater risk than other women of getting cancer. In an article in the *New Scientist* in 1978 Dr Joseph Hanion suggested that it would be impossible to prove conclusively for a few years whether chemical hair dyes are dangerous or safe. He did warn that ''hair dyes in general are so suspect that it must be the responsibility of the industry to prove safety''.

Most of the scientists involved in such tests are convinced of the connection between chemical hair dyes and cancer, but no conclusive research has been carried out to date. The British health authorities have decided to await positive evidence regarding the link between chemical hair dyes and cancer before legislation.

VEGETABLE HAIR COLOURS

By far the most effective of these is henna. In the critical tests carried out on hair dyes, henna came out with a clean bill of health, and it is known to be neither poisonous nor to cause skin allergies.

Henna is a greenish powder obtained from the crushed leaves and shoots of the shrub *Lawsonia alba (inermis)*. The best henna, usually called Persian henna, comes from Iran and gives a deep red colour. Egyptian henna is cheaper and gives a more orange colour. Chinese henna is less satisfactory as a hair dye, often containing twigs and bits ground into the powder; the quality of Indian henna varies widely.

Henna is excellent for hair. It conditions it, protects the ends from splitting and gives a glorious shine. It adds red colour to the body of your hair, with different effects depending on your own hair colour. On black hair it imparts reddish tones which will show particularly well in strong light. Brown hair becomes auburn and fair hair red. In all cases, henna fades gently over 2-3 months, thereby minimizing the effect of unsightly regrowth. It is unwise to use henna on very fair and very grey hair as the result will be orange. The most effective vegetable dye for fair hair is chamomile, which is used as a rinse or incorporated into shampoos and hair colours.

HENNA

Make sure you use pure henna. Any product which promises a complete colour change in 10-15 minutes is bound to be a compound. All processes using natural ingredients, including henna, take time to work. Equally, any smooth viscous liquid that pours beautifully from a bottle is unlikely to have much to do with pure henna, which is messy to use, smells like spinach and takes its time. If the product reacts to a previous hair colour or to a perm, it is also likely to be a compound.

Compound henna products are mixed with metallic salts or with aniline dyes and should be avoided. The addition of metallic salts reacts with previous hair treatments, such as perms, and the hair may split and eventually disintegrate. If the product is mixed with aniline dyes, the result is another chemical hair dye with its potential health risks.

We use Persian henna in our herbal hair colours and also sell pure Egyptian henna; you can make up your own mixes to produce the exact colour you want and have fun experimenting! For **darker tones,** mix 300ml of strong coffee with a packet of Egyptian henna and paint the paste over the hair. This will dull the red tones and give a darker hue. *Do not cover the hair* with a shower cap or foil. It is advisable to sit

HAIR COLOUR

Warning: explosives
Hydrogen peroxide mixes won't affect your health (though they may reduce your hair to the texture of straw), but they still pose potential dangers. *Never store* any unused mixture of lotion and powder as they are liable to explode in the container.

D.I.Y: beauty hint
Give a previous henna application a boost with a rinse: dissolve 50g of henna in 1.25 litre of boiling water, steep for 20 minutes, then strain. Use the liquid as a final rinse, collecting it in a bowl and pouring it over the hair several times.

Opposite: Healthy hair is strong hair, stronger than wire, strong enough to dangle an egg. Unkempt and neglected hair is weak and brittle, snapping at the slightest pressure.

in a steamy atmosphere as the circulating oxygen will slow down the red tones of the henna and allow the dark colour time to develop at a slower rate.

Henna can have a slightly drying effect, so if you have dry hair add 1 whole egg to the mixture before adding the coffee. As henna stains the skin, use rubber gloves when applying it; smooth cream on to the hair line, wiping off immediately any henna which spills over the hair line and on to the neck. Thoroughly wash hands, brushes, combs, sinks and any implements used. If you should happen to forget the time and launch into a lengthy telephone conversation, only to discover later a particularly virulent colour, *do not despair.*

In order to neutralize the vivid red colour you will need 50g turmeric, 50g rhubarb root, 15ml glycerine and 2 teaspoons alum. Mix all these ingredients, then slowly add sufficient hot water to make a creamy paste. Apply this all over the hair and leave for 20 minutes before rinsing it out. You can accelerate the process with an olive oil treatment: rub olive oil into the hair, use a hair dryer for 5 minutes, then wash the oil out. Repeat until the oil loses its reddish colour.

BODY SHOP HERBAL HAIR COLOURS
Our range of herbal hair colours is unique. They carry no health risk and can be used on top of other dyes and treatments. Hair coloured with them can be safely permed although a perm can take longer than usual to work. Herbal colour rinses are good for your hair and all will give added body as well as shine to the hair. The chart opposite shows which colours to use and which effect they will have on your hair. Follow the instructions on use and timing carefully. A cross on the chart means FORGET IT! Either it won't work on your hair or you will wish it hadn't!

Take into account the condition of your hair: the more porous it is, the quicker the colours will develop. The ends are always more porous than the roots so for an even colour always start by painting the mixture on to the roots, before treating the rest of the longer hair. Herbal hair colours will cover up to 25% grey hair, but as this is finer and more porous than the rest of your hair, the grey will take on a redder colour. These red highlights can look very pretty on dark hair, and on lighter hair they will turn golden-red.

A general rule on time limits: when first experimenting with herbal hair colours, it is a good idea to do a strand test and check the colour after the minimum time given in the chart. You can always leave it on for longer or re-apply it to deepen the colour, but it is difficult to remove the colour if it has been left on too long. Always go for the minimum time recommended for light hair; the darker your hair, the longer you can leave the colour. It is virtually impossible to overdo the length of time on naturally very dark hair; some people sleep with the paste on in order to develop the desired rich tones, at the same time ensuring marvellously conditioned hair. Do make sure to cover pillow cases with an old thick towel.

HERBS USED IN BODY SHOP HAIR COLOURS
Herbs work gradually, so be patient. Except for henna, all herbal rinses need time and repeat applications to achieve the desired effect. Exact shades cannot be guaranteed as they depend on the pigmentation of your hair, its condition and any previous treatments. **All herbal rinses are good** for your hair; they can be very attractive and it is fun to experiment with them.

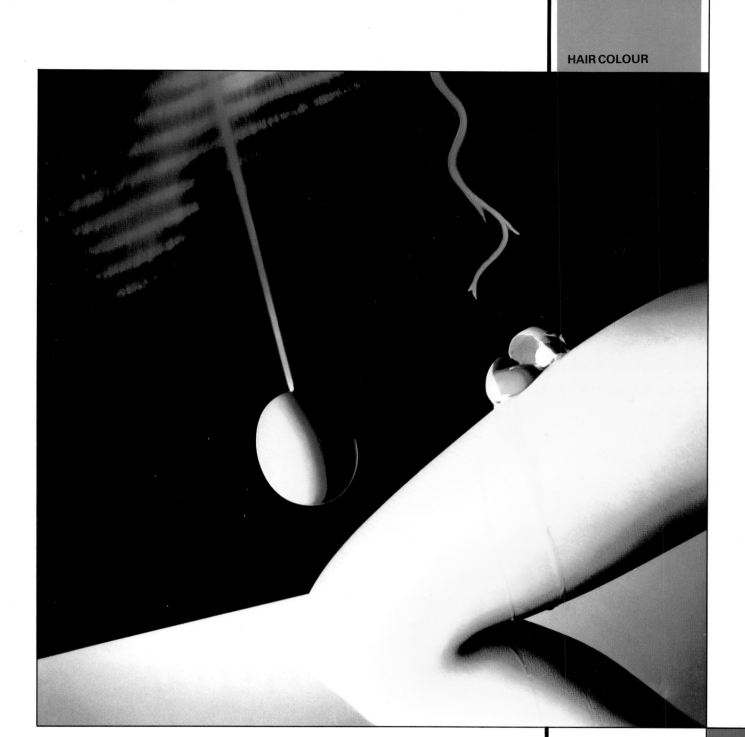

Myth or fact?
The use of walnuts to dye brown hair was first recorded in Roman times. The similarity in appearance between the walnut and the human brain fooled old herbalists into applying a cold compress of kernel skins to the head for brain complaints.

CHAMOMILE

This herb is valued for its natural lightening properties and as a colour improver of blonde hair. For a rinse, infuse 2 tablespoons of dried chamomile flowers in 600ml of boiled, hot water for ½-1 hour; strain and use the infusion as a final rinse, pouring it through the hair and collecting it each time in a bowl. Dry off in the sun.

For a brilliant conditioner and lightener, use one cup of dried chamomile flowers, 300ml of boiling water, the juice of 1 lemon and 2 tablespoons of henna wax. Steep the chamomile in the water for 30 minutes. Strain and add the lemon juice, then slowly stir the liquid into the wax. Smear the mixture on to hair and sit in the sun for as long as possible. Rinse out thoroughly.

For pale-ale colour to fading brown hair, steep 75g chamomile flowers in 300ml of boiling water for 30 minutes; strain and mix with 25g of henna. Paint the paste on to the hair and leave for 30 minutes. Rinse thoroughly and condition as usual.

RHUBARB ROOT

We use rhubarb root in our blonde herbal hair colour mix because it is the strongest of the natural lighteners. It brightens and lifts natural colours, giving them golden highlights. Rhubarb root takes effect on the first application, giving golden tones to blonde hair and chestnut highlights to dark hair. Mix 50g of rhubarb root with 600ml of white wine in a pan, cover with a lid and simmer gently for ½ hour. Cool and strain the liquid, then gradually stir in 1 teaspoon of kaolin to form a creamy paste. Apply this to the roots and comb through the hair; leave it on for ½-1 hour, depending on the porosity of your hair and on the desired effect. Rinse, shampoo and condition.

WALNUT

The colouring agent is extracted from the soft, unripe shells of walnut and promotes a rich dark hair colour. We use walnuts in Dark Brown Herbal Hair Colour to counter-act the reddish tones of the henna and to give a dark brown sheen to the hair. *Do not cover the hair* with a plastic bag or shower cap as walnut colouring works better when oxygen is allowed to circulate.

INDIGO

The colouring matter extracted from the Indigofera plant of India and Asia has been used for centuries to give a dark colour to hair. Persian women traditionally used henna to condition and give red highlights to the hair, then applied a paste of crushed indigo and water to darken it and give it a blue-black sheen. Indigo mixed with henna is known as henna reng and is used in our Dark Brown Herbal Hair Colour.

FACE

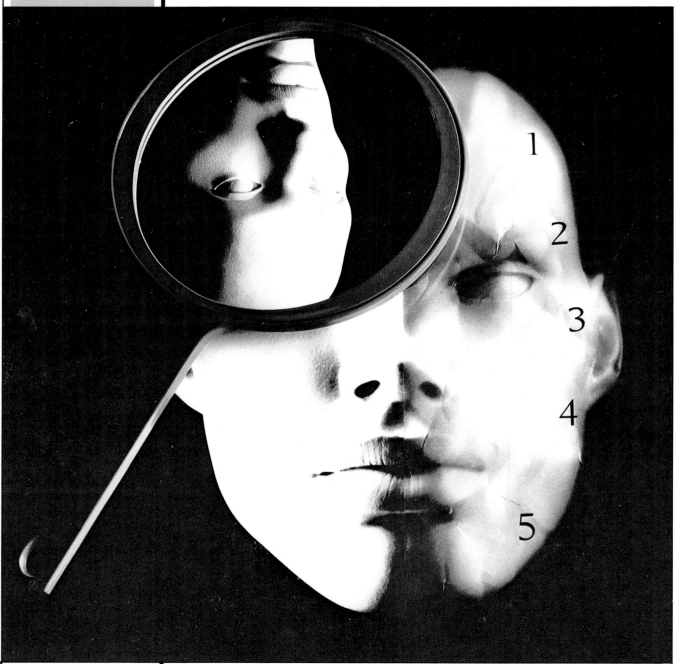

SKIN PROFILE

MOST SNAP JUDGEMENTS ABOUT PEOPLE ARE FORMED ON THE basis of their facial features. The eyes, said poetically to be the windows of the soul, are regarded as clues to the true character: closely positioned, they imply slyness; set wide apart they suggest honesty and directness. Thin mouths are equated with meanness, and full mouths with sensuality. Unconsciously we make such instant judgements, and they are made about us.

There is no hiding place for the face. Always exposed and vulnerable, it involuntarily expresses anger, fear, pain and shame, happiness, desire and joy, mirroring our every emotion. Precisely for that reason, a masked face evokes fear and horror: once the visual features are hidden, we cannot read or recognize the person, and fear of the unknown immediately arouses suspicion.

Consider then the cosmetic industry. It presents us with a huge paintbox of disguises, encouraging us to present a "normalized" version of ourselves by redrawing our features, redefining our shapes, evening out our blemishes. The ideal of beauty constantly before us is a mask behind which we can hide, a fashion face to put on, like expensive jewellery or couture dresses. Air-brushed, retouched and immaculate, the glossy adverts loom out as perpetual reminders of what we are not. The cosmetic industry creates needs we never knew we had and it survives on our feelings of inadequacy. Cosmetic surgeons make rich livings from cutting into faces in order to remould them into desirable images.

The time has come to redefine beauty: it is personal and individual, and we have finally begun to realize that beauty is also holistic: taking care of your health and skin is far more important than trying to change a feature.

Beauty begins with fitness and skin care, and you cannot expect a handsome painting if you disregard and maltreat the canvas. Skin care has become a boom industry, and men, too, are beginning to understand that dry, tight and sore skin, dull, lifeless and spotty, is neither necessary, healthy nor masculine. With the growing awareness of our environment, we also want to know just what we are putting on our skins, what effect they have, and whether the preparations are actually beneficial.

Scientists, cosmetologists, beauty therapists and consumers all agree that, broadly speaking, skin care does work. Or rather, that topical application of certain formulations of creams and lotions can cleanse the skin, help to alleviate acne, relieve dryness, making the skin more comfortable and smoother to the touch, softer and more attractive to look at, and help to delay, though not reverse, the ageing process.

There is a popular misconception that somehow "it's all the same stuff". It is not. There are hundreds, even thousands, of commonly used ingredients in skin preparations, some cheap, some expensive, some effective, some gimmicks, and price is not necessarily a proper guideline. Some products are long-established, others newly developed; some are well understood, others whose action, though

Fact: skin care products
Claims that all creams and lotions are the same are as silly as saying all food is the same. True, they serve identical functions, but they are composed of different ingredients with different properties, and some are more important than others.

Opposite: *The skin ages inexorably through time and, because it is constantly exposed to sunlight, the facial skin ages most rapidly. The process begins at birth and the clock can never be turned back. However, proper skin care will make it tick more slowly.*

Fact: skin moisture
Humid island climates bring out the best in skin. The Irish, British, Scandinavians, Polynesians and Fijians all have enviable skin.

effective, remains a mystery. Some formulas may be marvellous on one person and bring another one out in a rash; one of the best moisturising ingredients, for example, is lanolin, but a significant minority of people are allergic to it. Better formulations usually do mean better products, and the question constantly being asked is "are the most expensive products also the best?" The answer is no. There are only products which are the *best for your skin at any particular time*. As your skin and environment change over the years, so does the kind of most suitable skin product.

SKIN STRUCTURE

An understanding of the structure of the skin and the way in which cosmetics affect it is necessary in order to establish, first, which products will give the best results, and secondly, the cost-effectiveness of those products.

We have two kinds of skin, hairy and glabrous. Most of our skin is hairy, most profusely on the tops of our heads and least hairy on the female face. Glabrous skin is confined to the palms of our hands and the soles of our feet.

The skin is made up of layers of skin cells, the outer layers being known as the epidermis and the lower layers as the dermis. Cells are manufactured in the very lowest layer of the dermis and are gradually pushed closer to the surface as the top layers of the epidermis are shed. By the time the cells reach the upper layers they are completely dead. This process is known as the life-cycle of the skin and takes 21-28 days, older skin renewing itself more slowly. Skin cells are continually being shed from the surface of the epidermis, and up to 90% of household dust is dead skin.

The epidermis is the body's barrier against infection and virtually impermeable. It is comprised of several layers of closely packed horny cells, bonded and interlocked and known as the stratum corneum. Germs and bacteria can only penetrate this horny layer through injury; cracked dry skin, for example, is as much a health problem as a cosmetic one.

The dermis is the thicker underlying layer, containing all the important bits, whose fatty tissues act as a shock absorber of outside blows and as protection for the internal organs. The dermis is held together with collagen fibres, like bunches of twigs, and stretchy elastin tissue, which together form a structure for the cells, and is plumped up with fluid. Elastin maintains elasticity, and DNA (deoxyribonucleic acid) present in all cells, stamps out the pattern for new cell structures. Damage to the DNA by ultraviolet light causes permanent damage to the skin, because the DNA stamps out a different pattern. The dermis also contains blood, lymphatic and nerve cells, as well as sweat glands and hair follicles with their associated glands. Sebaceous glands secrete sebum which forms the major part of the skin's natural oil.

Two kinds of sweat glands in the dermis balance the pH value of the skin and help to wash oil and dirt from the pores. The apocrine glands, attached to the hair follicles, secrete a milky-white viscous substance, odourless at first but soon becoming a major factor in the development of each individual's personal scent. The eccrine sweat glands are widely distributed, often numbering as many as 600 per square centimetre of skin. They regulate body heat and respond to environmental temperature, emotional stress, ultraviolet light and rises in body temperature due to fever. They cause people of a nervous disposition to break out into a sweat.

The mixture of sweat and sebum forms a thin film known as the skin's acid mantle; this forms the skin's first line of defence against bacteria and infection. It has a natural pH of between 4.5 and 6, which should not be disturbed. It is irrelevant when some cosmetics and toiletries are claimed to be pH balanced because almost all creams and lotions are neutralized by the skin itself within one hour of being applied. However, soaps and detergents are alkaline-based and take much longer to neutralize; they must therefore be rinsed off properly from the skin.

SKIN TYPES

It is the activity of the sebaceous glands that determines your skin type, and you must assess what this is. Skin types are categorized as dry, oily, normal and combination. Normal skin is perfectly balanced, neither oily nor dry; it has become fashionable to label normal skin as combination, partly because it sounds more interesting, and partly because the average adult has slightly dry cheeks and a slightly oily zone around the forehead, nose and chin.

THE SKIN'S HIDDEN LANDSCAPE

Space technology has been adapted to study the profile of the skin, charting its peaks and hollows like a landscape on a foreign planet (see Ageing Skin). Close inspection of a piece of skin under a microscope reveals the inhabitants of the mountains and valleys as a whole population of different bacteria, happily co-existing and going about their daily task of making the skin safe for them to live on and for us safe to live in.

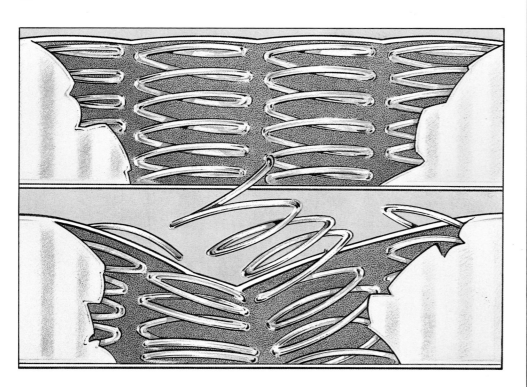

Young and old skin Young skin is like a firm new mattress. It is criss-crossed with tiny lines, plumped up with moisture and kept springy by collagen and elastin. As time passes these substances lose their strength: some of the lines grow weaker while others grow stronger becoming visible as wrinkles. The firm, soft mattress gradually becomes a worn, lumpy one: some of the springs have gone and the skin droops between those that remain.

DIY tip
Add Japanese Washing Grains to make a cleanser more exfoliating, particularly good through Honey Beeswax and Almond Oil. Rolled oats in cleansing cream work equally well.

Opposite: The three stages of skin care: clean dirt away with soap or with a cream or lotion cleanser; apply a toner to remove the last of the soap or cleanser and other grime; gently massage in a moisturiser to protect the skin.

The first step is the fairly steady action of what is known as desquamation. This is when the skin cells, born about 25 days earlier, have reached the surface and are being shed at the rate of about 4% a day. A second safety precaution is exerted by a whole colony of micro-organisms, such as bacteria, yeasts and bugs – up to seven million of them on the forehead alone. You acquire these organisms from your parents, or nursery nurse, in the first few days of life, and they stay with you for the rest of your life, forming a population which is as individual as a fingerprint. Most of them are harmless and do a good job destroying any harmful bacteria that land on the skin in the course of the day. A few are decidedly unwelcome, such as *Corynebacterium acnes*, which lurks in the follicles waiting to play a part in the formation of a spot. The related *Dermadex follicularum* hides in the follicles during the day and comes out at night to feed on everyone else.

You might think that as 4% of the skin is shed every day, and as bacteria and the acid mantle of the skin work together to maintain its protective layer, cleansing is neither necessary nor helpful. **Cleansing is the single most important aspect of skin care.**

Although harsh soaps can disrupt the acid mantle of the skin for a few hours, they make no impact on the bacterial population. The rubbing motion of soap and water, sponges or a granular product like Japanese Washing Grains all speed up the rate of cell renewal and make the skin look glowing and healthy. Helping to remove dead skin cells prevents the skin from looking grubby, sallow and dull, and clears the pore openings so that spots are less likely to form. Without thorough cleansing, it would take 25 days for make-up and city pollution to wear off.

The basic structure of the skin applies equally to all races, black, white and oriental. The only true difference between darker skins and paler ones is the amount of activated melanin. However, colour can affect your assessment of your skin type: black skin tends to look oilier simply because oil reflects better off a dark surface. Darker-skinned people may therefore assess their skins as oily and choose cosmetic formulations that are too harsh and degreasing. If you have dark skin and experience an irritant reaction from preparations for oily skins, change to a gentler formulation for normal skin and see if the condition improves.

CLEANSING

WE HAVE NO QUARREL WITH THE BEAUTY COUNCILLORS WHO intone the magic of cleanse, tone and moisturise for it is a very sound skin regime. We *do* question whether essential skin care should be pushed into the marketing arena as a concept of beauty and eternal youth, and we remain unconvinced that the promises attributed to specific formulas can be fulfilled. **Cosmetic creams affect the skin in so far as they cleanse, polish and protect it.** No more.

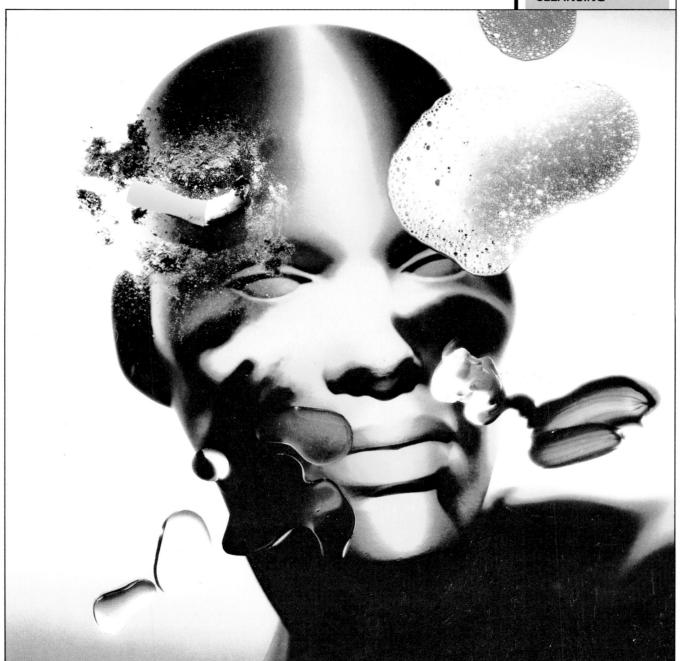

Cleansing the skin *is extremely rewarding: you instantly improve your appearance and there is no discomfort involved. Dissolve stale make-up by massaging cleansing cream over the face with your fingers. A natural sea sponge dipped into a soapless cleanser is ideal for removing make-up. For early morning cleansing spray on flower water and remove the excess with cottonwool.*

An almost mythical morality attaches to cleansing, and it is probably the only beauty routine universally approved of throughout the ages. The Victorians disapproved of vanity, but approved of the ancient Hebrew saying that "cleanliness is next to godliness". Harriet Hubbard Ayer, who strongly believed in women making the most of themselves, wrote in 1899: "the longer I remained in the laboratory manufacturing (cosmetics), the less I felt the average woman should use them, and the more respect I had for scrubbing brushes, soap and water, without other aids, at least for women under thirty".

The first known cleansing cream was what we today would call an all-purpose cleanser and moisturiser. It was invented by the Greek physician Galen in AD 150 and was a mixture of melted bees' wax and olive oil with water or rose-water beaten into it. He found that it gave a pleasant cooling sensation to the skin (hence the name cold cream), and also softened it far better than rubbing in olive oil. The scientific explanation is that oil in water or water in oil combinations preserve skin moisture more efficiently than pure oils.

Galen's cold cream was refined over the centuries, and olive oil was replaced with other oils which went rancid less quickly, such as almond oil. One widely used variant, rose-water ointment, otherwise known as Unguentum or *Ceratum refrigerans*, was made up by druggists until the turn of this century, and stored in ice boxes and cool places to be sold in small amounts. However, Galen's formula of oil mixed with water remains the basis of cleansing creams.

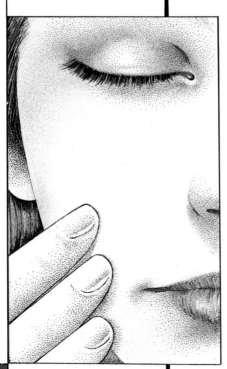
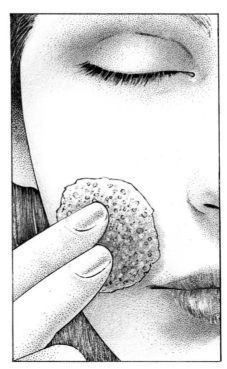
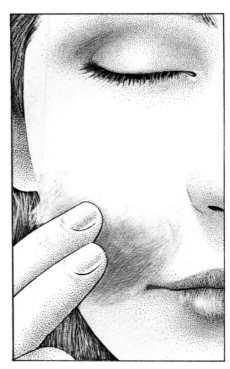

Meanwhile women were experimenting with other, less effective methods of cleansing. Soap, as always, went in and out of fashion. At one stage, water was thought to make skin sensitive to heat, cold and sunlight, and some women boasted of never having washed their faces. At the end of the 19th century Harriet Hubbard Ayer was giving women classes on how to wash their faces properly, instructing them to "take a scrubbing brush, dip into hot water, rub it vigorously with a cake of soap and bend over a bowl, and scrub the face with amazing vigor". One of her pupils commented that she "would as soon attack her face with a nutmeg grater."

Magic washing ingredients flourished through the ages, from Cleopatra and Poppaea who bathed in asses' milk, to Mary Queen of Scots, who occasionally washed in red wine for the sake of her complexion.

SOAP, FOR AND AGAINST

Soap is sometimes treated as a four-letter word! Objections to its use are three-fold. First, soap is ineffective in thorough removal of make-up and cannot deep-clean the pores; secondly, unless rinsed off thoroughly, the alkalinity in soap disrupts the acid mantle of the skin; thirdly, some soaps and detergent bars, or the perfumes in them, can cause irritation and sensitization.

Make-up should always be removed with a cream or lotion make-up cleanser. All make-up is wax or oil-based and needs a wax/oil combination to remove it. However, as it leaves a greasy film on the skin, this, too, must be

Exfoliation, the deliberate removal of dead cells, is one of the most effective ways of keeping skin looking young and can be achieved superbly and inexpensively by brushing with a facial brush, or by simply rubbing with a face flannel or even a potato. Facial brushing is especially good for black skins, because these shed their outer layers more quickly than white ones.

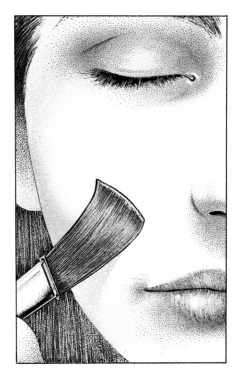

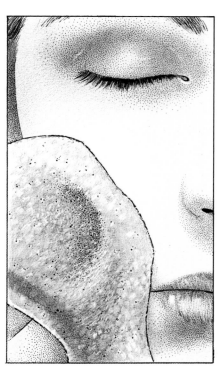

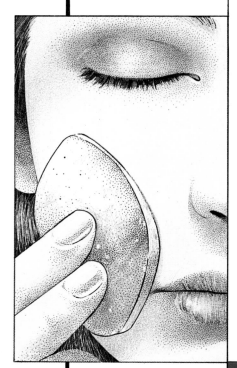

SKIN CARE AT A GLANCE

SKIN TYPE	CLEANSER	TONER	SOAP	MOISTURISER	NIGHT	SPECIAL TREATS	PROBLEM AREAS
SENSITIVE	Honey Beeswax	Honey Water	Milk and Protein Cleansing Bar	Sensitive Skin Lotion	Jojoba Oil Moisturiser	Honey and Oat Scrub Mask	Sage and Comfrey Open Pore Cream/ Camomile Aroma-therapy Oil
DRY	Orchid Oil/Honey Beeswax	Honey Water	Vitamin E Soap/ Jojoba Oil Soap	Aloe Vera Moisture Cream/Jojoba Moisture Cream	Carrot Moisture Cream	Honey and Oat Scrub Mask/ Wheatgerm Oil	
NORMAL/ COMBINATION	Orchid Oil/Honey Beeswax/ Cucumber Cleansing Milk	Elderflower Water	Orchid Oil Soap	Vitamin E Day Cream/Jojoba Oil Moisturiser/ Aloe Vera Moisturiser	Aloe Vera Moisturiser	Honey and Oat Scrub Mask/Japanese Washing Grains/ Almond Oil/ Jojoba Massage Oil/Rose/Neroli Aromatherapy Oils	Sage and Comfrey Open Pore Cream
OILY	Cucumber Cleansing Milk	Orange Flower Water	Vitamin E Clear Soap/ Lemon and Oat Facial Lather	Avocado Cream	Honey Beeswax Cleanser	Japanese Washing Grains/ Lavender Aromatherapy Oils	Sage and Comfrey Open Pore Cream

thoroughly removed. People who clean their skins with soap and water are following an excellent routine, provided that they cleanse off their make-up first with a cream or lotion and then remove the last traces of grease and grime with soap and water in place of a toner. Many dermatologists advocate this regime, particularly for oily skins. The alkalinity of soap is quickly neutralized by thorough rinsing and use of a toner and/or moisturiser.

The irritancy of soaps and detergent bars varies widely from brand to brand, and the most important question about soaps is not so much whether you should use them or not, but which soap to use. Ultimately you are the best judge of which soap is best for you. Indications that you use the wrong soap include a sensation of excessive tightening on the skin, drying and scaling and, in extreme cases, irritation, redness and sores. Dry or sensitive skins, and even normal skins, often experience such symptoms after washing with mass-produced soaps. They are often too degreasing for the fragile facial skin and have too high a perfume level for sensitive skins. Body Shop Jojoba Oil or Goat's Milk with Honey soaps are superfatted, with a high percentage of quality oils which will not dry out sensitive skins.

Oily or normal-to-oily skins can often tolerate, or even require, a strongly degreasing soap. Avoid superfatted or creamy soaps and change to a clear glycerine soap, such as Vitamin E soap or a syndet bar formulated for oily skins. It is well worth trying several soaps before deciding which is best for you.

FACIAL CLEANSING BARS

These are synthetic cleansers which can be used like soaps, but do not contain any actual soap. They can be formulated to be strongly degreasing and are therefore suitable for oily or acned skins. They are available as creams or as lathers for dry skins such as Glycerine and Oat Facial Lather, a grainy formula containing oats which help to clear away the dead cells which dull the complexion.

TIPS FOR WASHING

Avoid using very hot or very cold water on dry and sensitive skins as extremes of temperature can burst blood vessels and cause a red-veined look. Face flannels may also prove too abrasive and irritant as they may retain some of the detergent silicates with which they were laundered.

The best way of washing your face is to use your fingers, a well-rinsed sponge or a soft complexion brush. Black skins shed their outer layers slightly more quickly than white ones, and they particularly benefit from a gentle but thorough scrub with a soft complexion brush.

CLEANSING LOTIONS AND CREAMS

While soap and water make the skin look and feel clean, only cleansing creams and lotions are efficient enough to remove make-up properly. Unless the skin is thoroughly cleaned every night, it will look dull and lifeless, and will be more prone to spots and blackheads from clogged pores. Dirt and make-up also lodge in the crevices of the skin, working their way deeper in and encouraging wrinkles. A dirty carpet, apart from looking ugly, wears out quickly, because dirt and dust act as levers to increase the effect of everyday usage. In the same way, dirty skin looks drab and ages more quickly.

Tip: dry skin
Fashion models and peasant women alike swear by this remedy for dry skin: moisten the cleaned face with warm water, smooth jojoba oil over the face and splash with cold water. Finally, pat with face tissues.

Hint: exfoliating
The much maligned face flannel is an effective and inexpensive exfoliating tool.

DIY tip
A modern refinement of
Galen's original cold cream
cleanser:
Rose petal cleanser
4 tablespoons almond oil
20g bees' wax
3 tablespoons rose-water
(extra strength)
Melt the almond oil and
bees' wax in a *bain-marie*
until thoroughly blended.
Remove from the heat and
beat in the rose-water, drop
by drop, until the mixture
has cooled.

Opposite: *Plain water is
great for the skin and pores,
and a flower water is even
more refreshing to the skin.
Strong jets of water, from
showers, jacuzzis or from
wherever you can get
them, are both cleansing
and relaxing. Those with
sensitive skins should avoid
very hot or very cold water
because extremes of
temperature can burst
blood vessels and cause
thread veins.*

Cream or lotion remove make-up efficiently because the mixture of oil, water and waxes, when massaged on to the skin, melt and suspend particles of grime and cosmetics, freeing them from the skin. A cleanser with the right formulation will remove make-up and dirt, and if it is formulated for dry skin, for example, it will also leave a thin film of emollients. Cleansers like Honey Beeswax and Almond Oil Cleanser, for example, contain skin softening and moisturising ingredients like jojoba oil and honey, as well as cleansing almond oil.

Formulations for oily skins have different properties to help control excessive manufacture of sebum. Cucumber Cleansing Milk is a particularly gentle cleanser for oily skins and also suitable for delicate skins. The cucumber extract is the active ingredient in this product, while the cleansing oil is soya, a bland and non-reactive oil.

Cleansing and moisturising creams and lotions are all refinements of Galen's original formula. They have altered considerably since those early days of oil, waxes and water and most of those changes have little to do with cleansing the skin. They apply more to price, perfume and, more importantly, to the aesthetic feel of the product. Mineral oil replaced vegetable oil, at one-third of production cost, and because the natural colour of bees' wax was thought unattractive, it was bleached or replaced and Azo dyes added. Synthetic perfumes were also added. No changes in the cream's ability to cleanse were apparently ever contemplated.

TONERS

Toners are one of the original all-purpose perfumery and skin care products, sometimes known as waters or flower waters. They were mainly based on distilling ingredients suspended in water, some in simple recipes, others in complex manufacturing processes. In the 13th century, the Arabs mass-produced rose-water to such an extent that potentates pumped it through their fountains. Rose-water, one of the original ingredients in early classic Galen formulas for all-purpose creams, has been prized for more than 2000 years, and is still used today in many moisturisers, in "rose-water and glycerine" and in toners, as well as being an ingredient in perfumery. Unfortunately many of today's waters are synthetic; you can test the produce you are buying by shaking the bottle; if the water foams and the foam lasts for more than 30 seconds, the rose-water is likely to be synthetic.

Lavender water and orange flower water have equally long and venerable histories, as do waters with such glorious names as Virgin's Milk, Water of the Forty Thieves, Queen of Hungary Water, Water Without Equal, Water of English Lettuce, and ordinary flower waters, such as elderflower, jasmine, lemon, strawberries, etc. Virgin's Milk is the tincture of gum benzoin dissolved in water; it has gentle antiseptic properties and leaves the skin feeling soft and smooth. Our Honey Water is a mixture of Virgin's Milk, real rose-water and honey water.

Toners complete the cleansing process, removing the last traces of dead cells and grime from the skin. Depending on their formulation, they may also remove excess sebum from an oily skin, or soften and remove any residue of soap or cleanser. They often have a healing effect on a spotty skin and prepare all skins for the application of moisturiser, making it feel cool and refreshed. Toners with mildly acid ingredients, such as White Grape Skin Tonic, Elderflower Water and Orange Flower Water, also help to redress the skin's pH balance after the alkaline process of cleansing, thereby normalizing the skin's acid mantle.

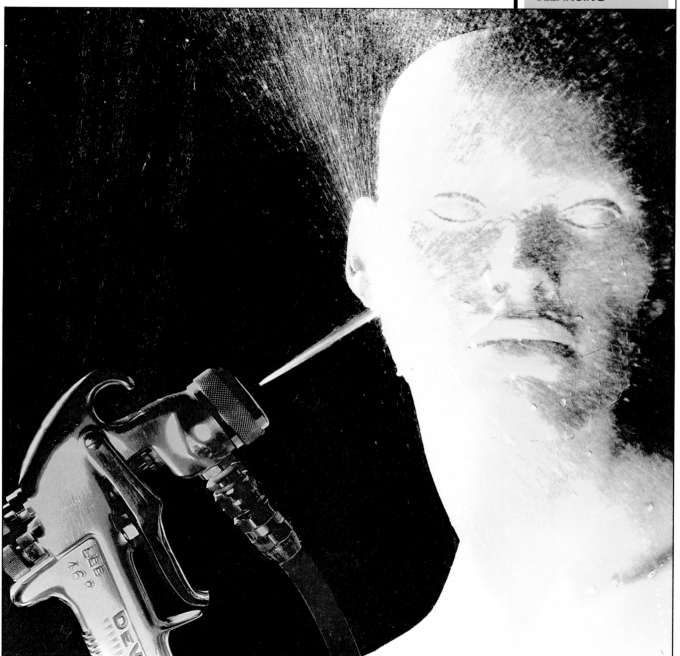

Myth breaker
An ancient remedy
professing to consist of
pure May dew gathered on
grassy banks of flowers and
promising extraordinary
powers of beautifying the
skin turned out to be a
mixture of orange flower
water, glycerine, borax and
distilled water – all well-
tried cosmetic ingredients.

PORES: AN OPEN AND SHUT CASE?

Toners are often misleadingly claimed to close the pores. This is a fallacy; the skin's pores do not open and shut according to some particular application. The only action which will tighten the neck of a pore opening is a swelling of the surrounding tissues. Large open pores are essentially hereditary, and the only way to ameliorate them is a sound skin care routine, which can keep them to a minimum. Pores which are allowed to become blocked with dead skin, sebum and grime can more easily become distended.

Nor will splashing with cold water close the pores; it merely gives the skin a feeling of coolness and tightness. Splashing alternately with hot and cold water can be damaging to the skin, as the rush of blood to the face may cause burst capillaries and a red-veined effect.

USING TONERS

Toners come under a variety of names, such as water, fresheners and astrigents. Many products described as fresheners are made from alcohol and water or water and glycerine, while those described as astringents usually have a higher proportion of alcohol. Astringents containing alcohol are unsuitable for dry and sensitive skins; if a particular toner dries your skin perceptibly, switch to a gentler preparation or a flower water. This applies particularly to black dry skin where alcohol may act as an irritant.

SKIN TONERS		
SKIN TYPES	**TONER**	**COMMENTS**
DRY/SENSITIVE	Honey Water	Contains no alcohol or colouring; made with oil of cloves, rose-water and honey, the latter being soothing and free from possible skin irritants. Ideal as a morning skin freshener
OILY/COMBINATION	White Grape Skin Tonic or Elderflower Water	Extract of grape is effective in removing dead cells; the acids restore the pH balance to the skin. Elderflower water has similar properties
ACNE	Honey Water	Honey has healing properties; the tincture of benzoin, which is also included, is antiseptic. Apply to the face with a spritz

Apart from providing the finishing touches to the cleansing routine, toners can be used as a gentle cleanser on their own, first thing in the morning when your clean skin needs only a gentle wipe, or as a quick clean-up during the day. Toners containing moisturising ingredients also have a gentle, softening effect, and can either prepare the skin to receive a moisturiser proper or be used during the day as a top-up if you do not wear make-up.

MOISTURISING

T HE WORD "MOISTURISER" COVERS A BROAD SELECTION OF creams and lotions which polish and protect the skin, keeping it soft, supple and comfortable. A moisturiser also helps to prevent the effect of drying, chapping and roughening caused by weather and other environmental conditions, like central heating and town pollution. Moisturisers also play a part in delaying the ageing of skin, although they can of course neither reverse nor prevent this.

It is now known that the amount of moisture, or water, in the skin is crucial to its appearance and health, making it soft, supple and firm. It is difficult to restore the lost moisture because the skin acts as a barrier; it supplies its own moisture and as long as the skin surface is in good condition it will prevent too much water from being lost from the lower layers.

Dry and cold weather dries out the upper levels of the skin, and the protective layer can then become brittle and cracked, exposing the lower levels to a greater risk of drying out. In extreme cases, the skin can rupture and even bleed. Moisturisers keep the skin supple by forming a film which prevents moisture loss and also protects it from dirt and grime. At the same time, some moisture is absorbed to interact with the top skin layers making it smooth and young-looking; certain vital ingredients, such as vitamins, can also have a beneficial effect on the skin.

In addition, moisturisers help to speed up the skin's renewal processes. In one particular test where the skin is stained with a dye visible only under a UV lamp, results show that skin rubbed regularly with a moisturiser renews itself more quickly than skin just rubbed. This test provides "proof" for the claim that certain moisturisers can rejuvenate the skin; they are usually in the expensive bracket, irrespective of the fact that *all* moisturisers have this same effect.

The effects of a moisturiser can be summarized as follows:

1. *forms* a film to prevent moisture loss and external damage.
2. *adds* some moisture to the skin, according to formulation.
3. The inclusion of active ingredients, such as vitamins, may have beneficial effects on their own account.
4. *speeds* up the skin renewal process.

Fact: cleansing
More than 83% of women under 65 use make-up regularly or occasionally (67% use it every day). However, 47% use a daily moisturiser, 44% a cleanser, 18% a night cream and 20% a toner. That means an awful lot of make-up isn't being cleaned off properly.

Fact: moisture
Moisture is the difference between a grape and a raisin.

Fact: moisturisers
Moisturisers supply a
protective cover to retain
the skin's own moisture,
like covering a swimming
pool to prevent evaporation
of the water by the sun.

Many sophisticated – and expensive – creams are not necessarily more effective than the simple ones based on Galen's original cold cream formula and those using natural ingredients like oil or jojoba oil. Lanolin is one of the earliest cosmetic ingredients and has exceptionally good water-absorbing properties. Basically wool fat, or the oil of sheep's fleece, lanolin is fairly similar to human sebum, and can mimic some of its qualities. Lanolin straight from the sheep has remarkable softening qualities and Australian sheep-shearers are said to roll on the shearing table at the end of the day in order to make their skin soft and supple. Lanolin has lost in popularity over the years because some people are allergic to it, but lanolin derivatives have been developed to crystallize the best properties of lanolin without the irritants.

Avocado oil is a relative newcomer to the cosmetics industry, although it was first incorporated in products in the United States in the 1930s. As it is rich in vitamins A and B and has good skin penetration properties, it is an ideal base for moisturisers for both oily and dry skins. Avocado oil has been used in the treatment of burns and on post-operative dressings. It also has valuable foaming and thickening qualities so that the inclusion of commercial thickeners and foaming agents can be reduced.

Spermaceti, an oil obtained from the sperm whale, was first used in cosmetic creams in 1780. Chemically it is neither an oil nor a wax, but it was marvellous for softening the skin and adding sheen to a cream. Until the sperm whale was declared an endangered species, thousands of whales were slaughtered indiscriminately and the oil sold at inflated prices. In the late 1970s it was discovered that jojoba oil had properties similar to those of spermaceti. It is a true and valuable newcomer to the cosmetic industry. The oil is extracted from the nuts of the jojoba shrub which grows wild in the arid deserts of Mexico and the Southern United States, and its moisturising qualities are excellent in that they are self-adjusting for all types of skin. Many commercial formulations use jojoba as a marketing tag, although it is often included in minimal proportions only.

The import of spermaceti and other whale products is now banned in Britain and other Western countries. Despite this, whales are still being killed. Japan does not observe the ban, and Japanese cosmetic products are not subject to any restrictions, nor are they obliged to list the ingredients.

NOURISHING CREAMS?

Moisturisers contain the most effective ingredients for improving the texture and quality of the outer skin layers. Other substances can also change and improve the skin. One is vitamins, others are the extracts of citrus and other fruits, including apples, grapes and apricots, and sugars. The latter promote healthy skin growth when applied in creams and toners because fructose contains active enzymes which help to speed up skin renewal and have some healing effects.

The skin is basically nourished by what we eat, and vitamins supplied through skin creams can in no way be a substitute for a healthy diet. However, vitamins have qualities of their own which are more healing and protective than nourishing. One of the vitamins in the B group is p-amino benzoic acid (PABA), much used in sunscreen products.

Vitamin A, which is essential for healthy skin and surface tissues, has proved useful in relieving dry skin and restoring its elasticity. The vitamin and its derivatives

Overleaf *"There is no
hiding place for the face.
Always exposed and
vulnerable, it involuntarily
expresses anger, fear, pain
and shame, happiness,
desire and joy, mirroring our
every emotion."*

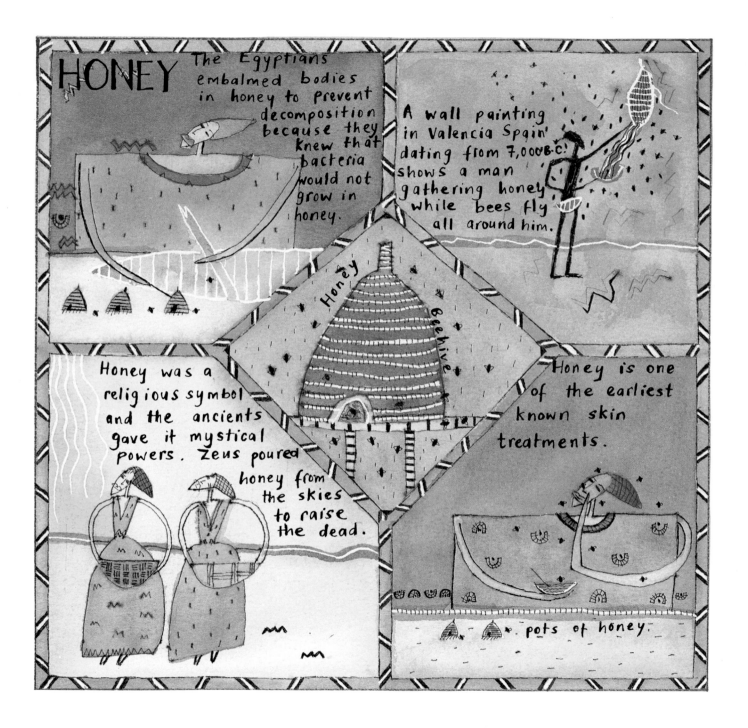

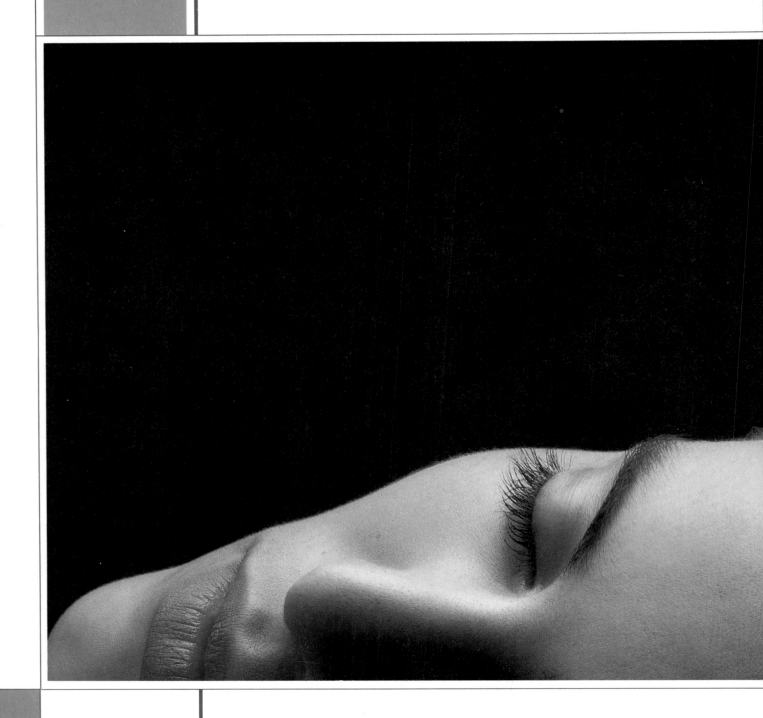

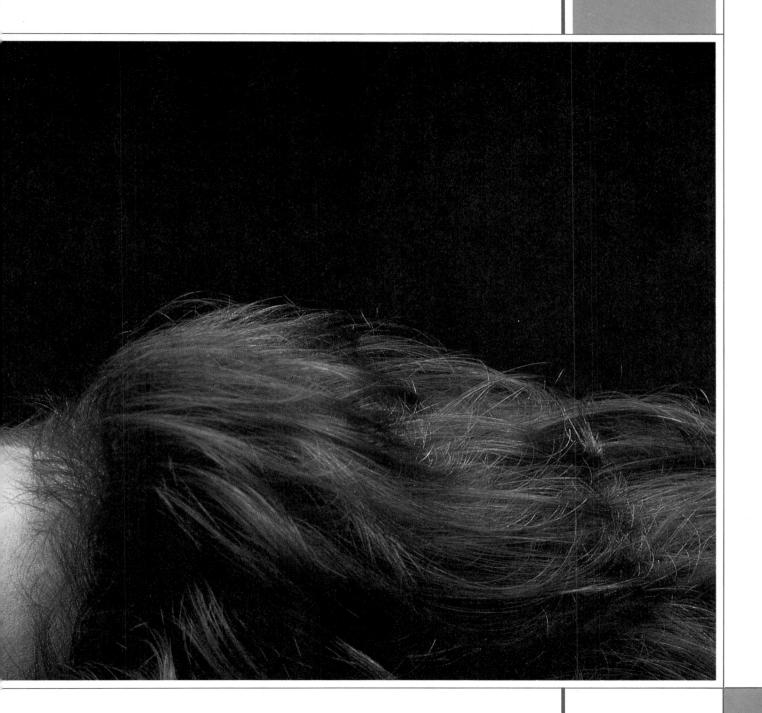

SHAVING

"There hath not come a razor upon mine head, for I have been a Nazarite unto God from my mother's womb. If I be shaven then will my strength go from me, and I shall become weak like any other man". Judges XVI 17-19

For many years before he started to use an open razor Samuel Pepys removed his beard with pumice. He was shaved once or twice a week by a barber.

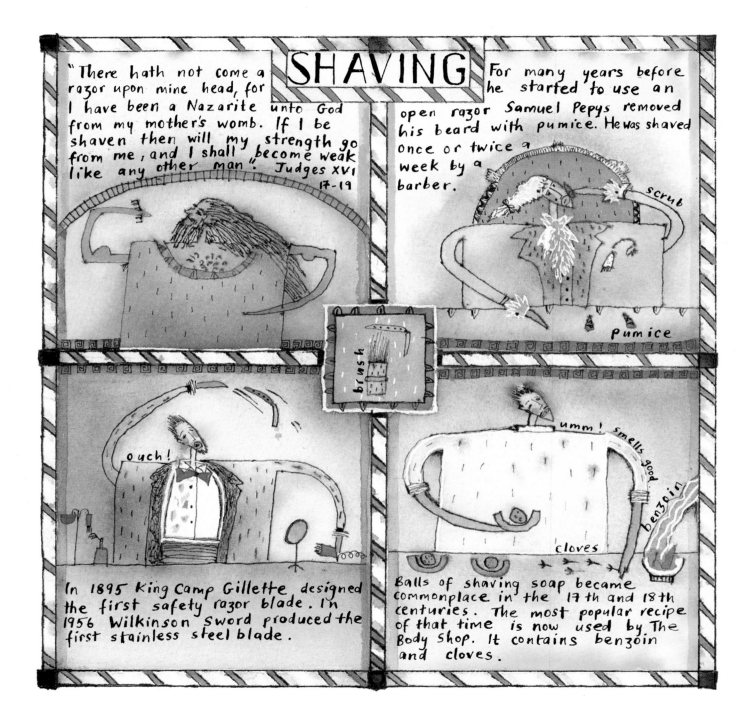

scrub

pumice

brush

ouch!

umm! smells good

benzoin

cloves

In 1895 King Camp Gillette designed the first safety razor blade. In 1956 Wilkinson Sword produced the first stainless steel blade.

Balls of shaving soap became commonplace in the 17th and 18th centuries. The most popular recipe of that time is now used by The Body Shop. It contains benzoin and cloves.

are also successful in the treatment of acne and for revitalizing normal skin and strengthening nails. The use of topically applied vitamin A is becoming more widespread in many skin care products, including our products like Carrot Moisture Cream and Facial Oil, and Neck Gel.

Vitamin E is another important vitamin in skin creams. It has been used to treat herpes and burns as well as to reduce the effects of scarring. It is said to improve the skin's absorption of substances, and the inclusion of vitamin E in a moisturising night cream gives the skin a better chance of absorbing vital moisture. Body Shop vitamin E products include Wheatgerm Oil, Vitamin E Cream and Rich Night Cream with Vitamin E.

USING MOISTURISERS

All skins need a moisturiser. Dry, normal and oily skin are all affected by wind and weather — as well as by central heating and air pollution. Dry skin in particular quickly becomes tight and flaky, chapping and reddening easily in winter and looking older before its time.

An expensive scientific study has come up with the startling conclusion that the best way to determine whether a cream was suitable is by the feel and effect of it on the skin. In other words, if it feels good, it is the right cream for you, and this will become apparent after a very few applications.

A moisturiser should be used twice a day; first thing in the morning and last thing at night, and also underneath make-up every time you apply it. Use gentle massaging movements because friction stimulates the supply of blood to the skin and encourages cell renewal. Gently massage the cream upwards or in small circular movements, on the forehead, from the chin up to the eyes, and up the "smile" line from mouth to nose. We also recommend applying moisturiser to slightly damp skin in order to seal in the water. *Never forget the throat in all face treatments; it shows the same telltale signs of ageing as the face.*

NIGHT CREAMS

Since Roman times night creams have been popular as anti-ageing remedies. Some were extremely inconvenient and sticky to use, and the French night cream of lanolin, vaseline and cold cream was not much better, especially as the mixture was smeared on to linen bandeaux and wound around the forehead and chin in the belief that the pressure of the bands would iron out the wrinkles.

Some kind of moisturiser should always be applied after cleansing; night time is a good opportunity to use a richer cream than would be convenient during the day. Recent dermatology research in the United States has revealed that different patterns of growth in skin and hair take place at night; this would suggest that creams may alter growth processes more effectively at night. On dry skin use a few drops of Wheatgerm Oil, on sensitive skin use Jojoba Oil Moisturiser and on normal skin use Aloe Vera Moisturiser.

Because the skin renewal cycle lasts between 21 and 28 days, it is necessary to allow a new skin care routine at least three weeks before results can be seen. If you are planning a new regime before a special event, such as a wedding or a holiday, start at least one month before, and once you have found a good system, take care to stick to it.

Tip: hair colouring
Use Rich Night Cream round the hair line before colouring with henna, to prevent staining of the skin.

*Opposite: Gels have an
advantage over lotions in
that they do not become
runny in hot atmospheres
or summer heat. For the
eyes we recommend a
transparent gel which cools
and refreshes the eye area,
and is especially soothing in
smoky environments or on
long air flights. For the lips,
a creamy gel to protect
them from sun and wind.
For the neck, an opaque gel
with orchid and carrot oils
to smooth and soften the
skin.*

LIP CARE

Lips need different products from the rest of the face because they contain no sebaceous glands but more melanin. Extra melanin helps to protect them against sun, but not against the drying effects of wind and cold.

Cracked and chapped lips, apart from looking unattractive, are particularly vulnerable to bacterial infection. Many people who do not otherwise suffer from sensitive skin find that bright sunlight or extreme weather conditions bring their lips out in sores or herpes. Most lips can be protected with one or two daily applications of a good lip salve, like Body Shop Lip Balms, but if you suffer from sun-reactive sores you will need a lipsalve with a built-in sunscreen. Castor oil and honey are both good lip soothers, although the temptation to lick off the latter may mitigate its effectiveness. For herpes, try Camomile and Eucalyptus Aromatherapy Oils, both of which have been successful in alleviating cold sores and herpes.

Masks and exfoliating scrubs should not be taken down to the lip area, but facial massage with oils is as beneficial to lips as to the rest of the face. Consult your doctor on any lip sores which do not clear up within a few weeks.

EYE CARE

The fine skin around the eyes is the first to show wrinkles and bags because it is the thinnest skin on the body (0.5mm or roughly the thickness of an airmail envelope), and because it has no oil glands. The eye areas need special care, and the choice of a suitable cream or oil is particularly important because it is so close to the mucous membranes of the eyes.

It is essential to remove eye make-up thoroughly with a special cleanser. Never pull and tug at it with soap and water. Body Shop cleansers, such as Cucumber Cleansing Milk, Honey Beeswax, Almond Oil, and Orchid Oil, can be used to remove eye make-up, and all traces of the cleanser itself must be thoroughly removed. Thereafter, gently pat Wheatgerm Oil or Elderflower Eye Gel into the tissues around the eyes; avoid using too much gel or oil as stinging results from over-generous application. Heavy creams will make the eyes puffy and baggy in the morning; during the day use a little light foundation or moisturiser around the eyes; never powder as it cakes around the wrinkles and accentuates them.

Natural eye brighteners include slices of cucumber or cold tea bags over the eyes while resting. However, if you have sensitive eyes the latter will make you look as if you had been crying for a week. The Body Shop Coolpacs are also refreshing as an eye treatment. In general, eyes have their own effective cleansing mechanisms, and medicated eyedrops should not be used on a regular basis.

COSMETICS AND CONTACT LENSES

You can still use cosmetics with contact lenses, but take the following precautions:

1. Insert lenses before applying make-up.
2. Never apply hand cream just before inserting the lenses and never use oils round the eyes — both will form a film over the lenses.
3. Don't use lash-building mascara; the fibres may become trapped in the lenses and cause irritation.
4. Keep eyes closed when hairspray is used.

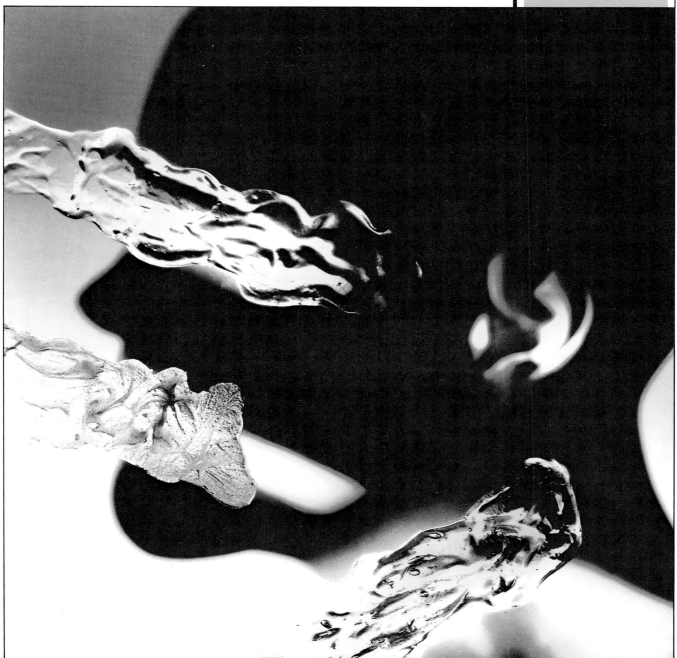

Tip: face masks
Astringent face masks can be drying for sensitive skins; mix with some of your usual moisturiser before applying the mask.

TREATS FOR THE FACE

PECIAL TREATMENTS FOR THE FACE ARE INVALUABLE, AS PICK-ME-ups when you feel or look particularly tired, and as regular weekly treatments with long-lasting benefits to the skin. They fall into three categories: exfoliation, masks and massage.

EXFOLIATION

Literally meaning shedding of surface tissues, exfoliation removes the top layer of dead cells from the skin. It goes in and out of fashion as much as soap and water, yet it is the oldest known beauty treatment, probably one of the most effective and one which receives unanimous support from dermatologists. Exfoliation was mentioned in one of the oldest medical documents ever found, an Egyptian papyrus roll from 1500 BC which included a recipe using meal of alabaster, water from the qebu plant, fresh abt grain, honey and human milk to be rubbed over the face. Another recipe, with the equally unfamiliar ingredients of cremar gelanthi, saponin and pulverized pumice, was in use as late as the turn of the 19th century.

Favourites that have stood the test of time include oatmeal rubs, and scrubbing with pumice stone, loofahs and granules; many of today's exfoliating products are formulated to perform similar functions. In the opinion of dermatologists, thorough exfoliating removes surface oil, dead cells and dirt, loosening acne plugs and black-heads. It also makes scaly, reddened and sun-damaged skin look cleaner and gives normal skin a healthy glow from the acceleration of circulation and cell renewal, both of which improve the skin's texture. Exfoliaton, which has been used in the treatment of extreme skin conditions such as psoriasis, is particularly beneficial for black skins and for restoring the flow to ageing skin.

Exfoliation is a forceful treatment, and it is important to choose the right method for your skin type. Oily and acned skins need thorough exfoliation, while dry and more sensitive skins become inflamed and irritated with too powerful a product; this is especially so with black skins which scar more easily than white skin after over-rough removal of spots and blackheads.

Rub dry skin with a few drops of Jojoba or Carrot Oil, then rub with a teaspoon of Japanese Washing Grains. Scrubs, such as washing Grains, really come into their own for oily or spotty skins. Remove make-up and put a teaspoon of the grains in the palm of the hands; mix them with a drop of water and gently massage it into the oily areas and over clogged pores. Rinse off with luke-warm water.

MASKS

Masks also have an exfoliating effect, gently lifting dead cells off the skin surface, and often having moisturising or other active properties; the enzymes in fruit masks, for example, do tighten and brighten the skin. Masks are less abrasive than exfoliant scrubs and are therefore more suitable for very fine dry and sensitive skin, for broken veins and for skins in the first stage of ageing. The Body Shop Honey and Oat Scrub Mask is more a mask than a scrub; smooth it over a clean face and leave it to dry for five minutes, then rinse it off with a damp sponge. Even better, apply a mask while you soak in the bath.

HOME-MADE MASKS

Many kitchen ingredients can be used for effective masks, with little trouble and at little expense. Yoghourt, fresh or sour cream and butter all make excellent bases for masks for dry and dull skins. Mash fresh peeled apricots with a little olive oil and cream, or squeeze ripe strawberries and a small lump of butter to a paste. Mashed peaches, bananas or grated apples can be mixed with honey, cream or yoghourt, and on their own honey, plain yoghourt, cold porridge and strawberries all make good home masks. Rinse them off with cool water.

Shape a piece of cheesecloth or butter muslin to fit the face and the front of the neck, cutting holes for the eyes, nose and mouth. Immerse it in warm oil (try Body Shop Jojoba Oil or Apricot Kernel Oil), or honey for dry skins and in milk or iced astringent lotion, such as Orange Flower Water or White Grape Skin Tonic, for oily and dull normal skins. Place the mask over face and neck, with eye pads over the eyes and leave for 10-20 minutes; carefully peel off the mask and wipe the skin clean. Spray the face with a tonic lotion and let it settle for a few minutes before applying make-up.

MASSAGE

Particularly beneficial to dry and ageing skin, massage stimulates circulation and makes the skin more supple. Harriet Hubbard Ayer firmly believed in the power of massage to smooth out wrinkles, although she also believed that the presence of many wrinkles was a question of morality and character, and that gossip, vengeful-ness and petulance all etched their own particular lines.

Modern dermatologists would be inclined to say that no wrinkles, vengeful or not, could be smoothed out, but massage still has many benefits. One of the best anti-wrinkle treatments is foot massage – and well-fitting shoes – because painful feet cause the face to screw up! You can treat a friend to a relaxing facial massage or pamper yourself while you laze in a hot bath when the steam will help the skin to absorb the oils. The art of facial massage established in Sweden in the 1890s is still the recommended method. Basically, it consists of upward semi-circular gentle strokes along the lines of the muscles, up over the jawline to the mouth and out over the cheeks, from the centre of the forehead to the temples, above the eyebrows and below the eye sockets to the sides.

Facial oil such as Apricot Kernel Oil or Wheatgerm Oil is suitable for very dry or prematurely ageing skin, and Sweet Almond Oil or Jojoba Oil for normal or sun-dried skin. Massage gently for about 15 minutes. Lavender Aromatherapy Oil, antiseptic and regenerative, is ideal for oily skins, while a mixture of Neroli and Lavender is worth trying on acne scars. To give your face a treat, massage it with plenty of Jojoba or Carrot Oil. Next take a teaspoon of Japanese Washing Grains and gently massage into the skin. Wipe off oil and grains and then hold the face over steaming water for five minutes. Dry and apply Honey and Oat Scrub Mask. Relax and let the mask dry. Remove mask and freshen up with a spray of Honey Water.

Tip: home-made scrubs
Oatmeal and ground almonds both have degreasing effects, beneficial to oily or acned skins.

Honey and almond cleanser:
1 tablespoon honey
1½ tablespoons ground almonds
milk
Combine the honey and ground almonds with enough milk to make a paste. Rub well into the skin; rinse off with cold water.

Grapefuit and oatmeal scrub:
juice of a grapefruit
3-4 tablespoons oatmeal
Blend the grapefruit juice and oatmeal to a fine paste; smooth it on the face as a mask for 15 min; remove with warm water, scrubbing the abrasive oatmeal into the skin. Rinse off with cool water.

Tip: oily skin
A facial massage with lavender oil is beneficial for oily skin; remove all traces of oil with moist cottonwool.

Tip: for spots
Wash your face with clear glycerine soap and gently massage it with one teaspoon of caster sugar; rinse thoroughly. Spots seem to beat a retreat within 10 days.

A spot is created when a sebaceous gland is upset causing thickened sebum that mixes with grime and dead skin cells to block the mouth of a pore. Bacteria multiply beneath the blockage, causing an infection. Gradually dead bacteria and white corpuscles are squeezed upwards like toothpaste from a tube. Spots and acne are difficult to prevent because there are numerous possible causes of an upset sebaceous gland. Dirt is rarely a cause but it can exacerbate the problem. Acne-prone skin should therefore be protected from both dirt and grease, but don't wash too often and don't use too oily a soap: three times a day with a simple soap is best.

ACNE

THIS IS PROBABLY THE MOST DISTRESSING COMMON SKIN CONdition, and while it is considered a teenage affliction, it can be problematic in the twenties and thirties. Acne is virtually unknown in children; it develops in the early teens, reaching its peak in girls at the age of about fourteen and in boys at about sixteen and usually continues for several years afterwards. The worst aspect of acne is the effect it has on the sufferer's confidence. While dermatologists do not regard acne as a "nervous disease" as such, it is often accompanied by depression and anxiety, and the resulting nervous gestures, such as niggling away and picking at spots, can lead to scarring and apparent resistance to treatment.

Acne occurs on all kinds of skin — black, white and oriental - although one dermatologist has observed that he considers American teenagers to be the worst afflicted. There would not appear to be a single common cause for acne and its severity is the result of many intrinsic factors.

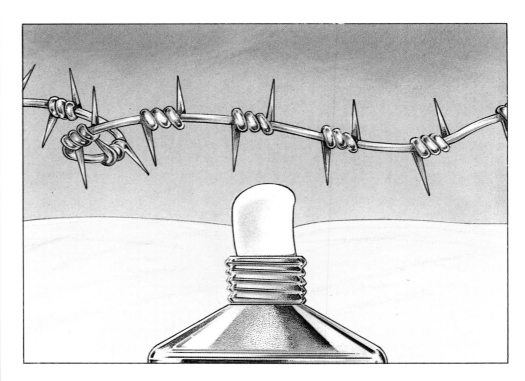

SPOTS AND BLACKHEADS

A spot starts with a disturbed sebaceous gland. In certain skins, the normal hormones upset the sebaceous glands, causing redness and irritation; the sebum thickens and becomes mixed with grime and the debris of dead skin cells at the sides of the hair follicle or pore, blocking the mouth of the pore. In the dark, airless follicle beneath, bacteria start to multiply, while the surface of the blockage oxidizes at exposure to air and turns black; from the outside this appears as a blackhead.

Eventually the spot ruptures – or is ruptured by picking – and the infected material of dead bacteria and white blood corpuscles is disgorged over the skin, some of it also spreading through the walls of the skin. There is some evidence that regular sufferers have "acne-permeable" skin, more likely to be penetrated by irritant materials. As with the common cold, there is no perfect cure for acne, only certain preventive measures.

CONTROLLING ACNE

A lot of needless guilt is often associated with acne and there is a common misconception that acne is somehow an "unclean" disease. Such unsympathetic attitudes do little to help the sufferer to understand and control acne. Over-zealous washing can be an exacerbating factor because soaps which are frequently suitable for regular use two or three times a day may irritate the skin when used six or seven times daily.

Washing is a fairly superficial action and does nothing to unplug the pores or penetrate into inflamed follicles. However, as acne is due to increased sebum production, it is sensible to keep the skin's level of oiliness down to a sensible minimum by using the right types of soap and cleanser. Wash two or three times a day with a soap designed specifically for oily or acne skin, like transparent glycerine Vitamin E Soap. It is important to use a simply formulated soap as some acne may be inflamed by perfumes or superfatted agents; baby soaps and richly lathering creamy soaps, suitable for dry skin, are definitely bad for acne sufferers.

COSMETIC-INDUCED ACNE

Another popular misconception relates to make-up; teenage girls are frequently told that their acne is caused by "all the stuff they plaster on their face". This is largely inaccurate. A type of cosmetic-induced acne, known as *Acne cosmetica*, strikes women in their 20s and 30s whose teenage acne had largely cleared up. *Acne cosmetica* is always mild and nearly always chronic. It is chiefly a reaction to certain cosmetic ingredients, such as lanolin, petrolatum (petroleum jelly) and some essential fatty acids.

Colour cosmetics are not responsible for *Acne cosmetica*, nor is excessive use of blushers or lipsticks; the culprits are found in moisturisers, foundations, night and suntanning creams which contain benzophenone. If you have sensitive acne, always check that suntan products contain no benzophenone, if necessary by writing to the manufacturer. Body Shop products do not contain benzophenones. If you suspect mild but persistent spots are due to *Acne cosmetica*, try cleansing with Body Shop Honeyed Beeswax or Almond Oil Cleanser and wipe it off with damp cottonwool.

Acne cosmetica can take 6-8 months to clear up, so avoid changing from one cream to another. However, if more spots appear after treatment with a particular

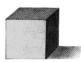

Fact: beauty aids
Patches, originally designed to cover spots and smallpox scars, became fashionable beauty aids. Some were placed by the eyes to make them appear larger, others as coquettish trivia by the nose, and patches on either cheek denoted the wearer's politics.

Fact
Dr Kligman, the American dermatologist, has found after exhaustive tests that skin *cleansers do not cause acne*. Sufferers, however, are advised to stick to soap and water cleansing.

Tip: sensitive skin
Mix Honeyed Beeswax with Washing Grains for a deep cleansing mask which exfoliates sensitive skins without drying them.

Warning: Beatle forehead
The long, over-the-forehead hairstyle, popular in the 1960s, led to a near-epidemic of forehead acne among young males.

Sun and tobacco smoke
both hasten the ageing of the skin. The sun's ultra-violet rays damage it and dry it out. The skin of smokers is known to wrinkle and age years sooner than that of non-smokers. The benzopyrene present in tobacco smoke inhibits the body's absorption of vitamin C, thus damaging healthy collagen. It causes the blood vessels in the skin to contract and inhibits circulation.

cream, **stop it at once.** Spots do not "come out" from cosmetic treatment, but they can be induced if strongly medicated ingredients irritate the surface of the skin; this causes puffiness which in turn closes the mouths of the pores resulting in yet more spots and blackheads.

DIET

The skin, like the rest of the body, reflects your diet and general living pattern; it needs an adequate supply of proteins, minerals and vitamins in order to stimulate and maintain healthy growth. However, beyond that generalization it is difficult to determine how much effect diet has on acne. A Body Shop study on acne patients showed that on a strict macrobiotic diet and with herbal remedies to drink, there was a pronounced improvement, but otherwise dietary changes had little effect on acne. Tests carried out in the United States confirm that an extreme low-fat diet has some effect, but that the exclusion of decidedly unhealthy and fatty foods like chips and chocolate make little difference to the severity of acne.

Other studies indicate that a rash of spots after an illicit chocolate bar may be related to tension and guilt. On the other hand, it was found that Eskimos did not suffer from acne until they were introduced to chocolate along with other aspects of Western life. The inter-related causes of acne are extremely complex; some sufferers may notice a marked benefit from cutting down on dairy foods, so this is well worth trying.

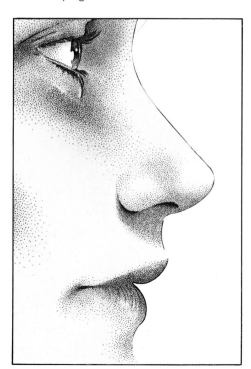

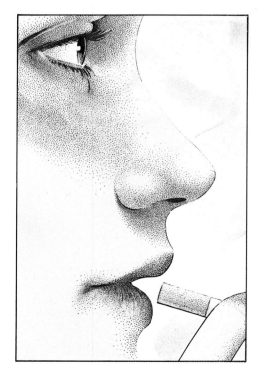

PICKING AT SPOTS

Many old wives' tales are based on facts, and scientific investigation endorses that if you pick your spots, you will spread them and leave scars. The infected material on the surface is spread by the fingers, and the pressure disperses it through the skin walls, especially in acne-permeable skin. However painful and unsightly, **leave spots alone** or cover them with cooling and soothing topical remedies to lessen the discomfort.

One particularly disfiguring type of acne, called Excoriating Acne, is usually only found in very disturbed teenage girls. Their self-destructive impulses lead them to pick and attack their spots constantly, turning what might have been a mild case of acne into a virtually untreatable disease. The spots spread quickly, leading to scarring. The disease can be as serious as *Anorexia nervosa* and requires psychotherapy before clinical treatment of the acne can hope to succeed.

Various habits and body postures can help to spread acne. People who study or consistently watch television with the same part of their face resting on their hands may find that acne recurs more often in exactly those places. Stress and nervous gestures, such as rubbing the face with the fingers can have the same effect. The best way to alleviate stress-induced acne is to desist from such gestures.

Equipment like chinstraps, motorcycle helmets, faceguards and sweatbands, and clothing like hats, turtleneck sweaters and shirt collars can also be responsible for increasing acne on those parts of the face and neck they repeatedly touch.

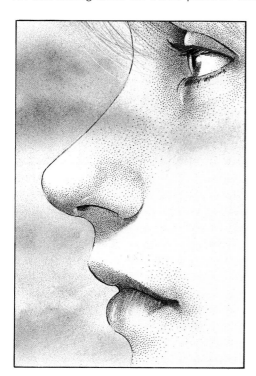
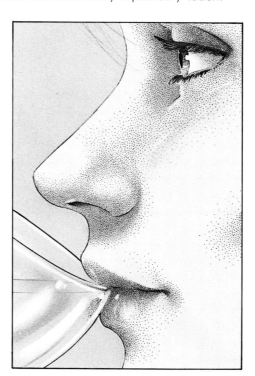

ACNE

Fact: ''organic'' cosmetics Chemically, a substance is said to be organic if it has a carbon compound, whether natural or synthetic. Among millions of items, vaseline, vinegar and silk contain carbon as do most creams, oils and lotions.

City air and alcohol *are also detrimental to healthy skin. The dirt, smog and grease of the city must be kept at bay with a regular and effective cleansing routine. Alcohol contains none of the vitamins or minerals essential for cell growth. It stimulates the appetite, thereby provoking overeating; robs the body of B vitamins; and ruptures blood vessels causing a network of broken veins on the face.*

Opposite: Aerosols are unnecessary and contribute to the destruction of the environment. They are expensive to manufacture and therefore to buy, and contain a substance which floats up into the atmosphere to gradually erode the all-important ozone layer. They cannot be refilled and become rubbish as soon as they are empty, adding to the debris of the disposable era. A bottle, on the other hand, can be refilled an infinite number of times, and its contents can be poured into an atomiser to create a non-polluting spray.

TOPICAL TREATMENT

Topical treatments (topical means applied to the skin) are effective against acne and spots, provided that you choose the right remedy. A sensitive skin with only a few spots or mild acne may well finish up with more spots after treatment with a harsh exfoliant or scrub because the ingredients have set off further inflammation and irritation. A mild scrub like Body Shop Honey and Oat Scrub Mask is preferable for such cases. Oatmeal is a traditional gentle abraser and the other exfoliating ingredient, kaolin, gently draws out impurities. Dermatologists regard exfoliation as particularly important in acne treatment, removing deep down impurities and helping to unplug blocked follicles.

On strong acne and oily skins, use a product like Japanese Washing Grains; the finely sieved, ground aduki beans clear clogged pores. Always use scrubs or exfoliants *before* applying specific acne treatment creams.

A number of over-the-counter spot remedies are readily available, but unless you choose one appropriate to your skin, you may start a secondary inflammation or another spot. Two currently popular ingredients for spot treatments are retinoic acid (vitamin A derivative) and benzoyl peroxide, the latter sometimes considered inflammatory though effective.

The Body Shop Sage and Comfrey Open Pore Cream has a mildly exfoliant and healing effect. It contains comfrey, which relieves inflammation and heals skin eruptions, and allantoin, which heals lesions by removing unwanted tissue; it is an important ingredient in treating wounds. The other two active ingredients, sage and witch hazel, both have astringent and cooling effects which help to remove the temptation to pick and burst spots.

DRUGS AND SURGERY

In extreme cases of acne, doctors will prescribe a course of antibiotics, which are usually effective. However, antibiotics are best kept to a minimum in order to prevent resistance from developing. Pre-menstrual acne often improves with the use of the contraceptive pill, though it usually takes about five cycles to show up.

SKIN ALLERGIES

KIN SENSITIVITY AND ALLERGIC REACTIONS HAVE INCREASED IN line with pollution of the environment and stress in our daily lives. Allergic reactions to cosmetics are surprisingly low, and studies on external irritations and their effects on the skin showed that cosmetics and toiletries were responsible for only 6% of the problems.

Environmental factors can trigger off a number of allergies. In any one week your skin may come into contact with soaps, detergents, washing-up liquids, bath oils, toothpastes, skin creams, shampoos and conditioners, suntan lotions, talcum

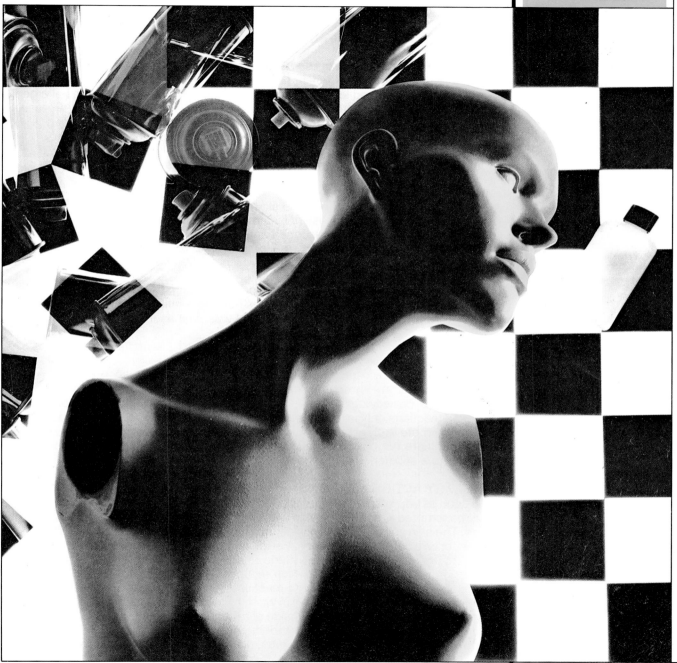

Fact: on glycerine
Products with a high glycerine content work best in humid climates because they draw moisture from the air. In dry climates, the effect is reversed: glycerine draws moisture from the skin.

Dark skins contain more melanin than fair skins and are therefore less prone to wrinkles. However, despite their higher concentrations of melanin, both the Mediterranean and negroid skin-types dry up and wrinkle with prolonged exposure to the sun.

of the highly magnified skin profile, a technique known as profilometry, shows a young, glowing and elastic skin to be almost jagged in the way pockets of moisture form peaks and hollows.

As the skin ages it "flattens" and looks duller. Some of the tiny lines grow weaker, others stronger as the collagen and elastin become weaker and less well distributed; the criss-cross pattern disappears, to be replaced by other, stronger lines, either at random or running in the same direction. *These are wrinkles.* The skin begins to resemble a lumpy mattress no longer evenly supported on a mesh of springs: some of the springs have gone and the fabric appears to droop between the peaks. The magnified skin profile shows a flat surface which reflects less light and therefore appears dull.

FACTORS IN SKIN AGEING

Several factors are responsible for the different rates at which skin ages: heredity, extreme weather conditions, stress, diet, etc, but the primary reason for premature ageing of the skin is the damage done by the sun's ultraviolet rays. Sunlight damages both DNA and elastin, drying out the skin, and this occurs every time the skin is exposed to sun. Your face, neck and hands are the first to show signs of age because they are most often exposed.

The damage done by the sun to the skin's elastin, collagen and DNA is irreversible and cumulative. It begins on day one of your life and tots up like a bank overdraft; you

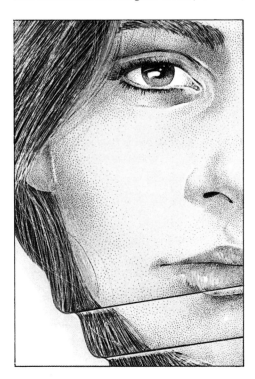

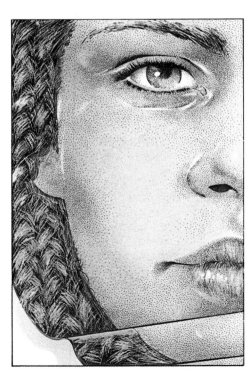

will have to pay up sometime, but proper skin care can insure that you pay later rather than sooner.

In 1980 the Chief Dermatologist of Massachusetts General Hospital, Dr Thomas Fitzpatrick, told the scientific community that "sun is one of the four deadly pleasures in life, the others being alcohol, nicotine and food". The greatest favour you can do to your skin is to avoid sunbathing altogether. You may think that two or three weeks in the sun once a year will hardly affect your skin, but while such exposure will hardly encourage skin cancer, it will accelerate the ageing process. Dr Lorraine Kligman, an eminent research dermatologist, has presented convincing evidence that prominent wrinkles would result over two years from sunbathing for only two hours daily during July and August.

Studies have shown that 85% of UVA rays, which are those responsible for premature ageing, can penetrate window glass, 70% a car windscreen, and some can penetrate clothing, particularly nylon. UVA rays are at their fiercest during summer, but they are also transmitted and reflected during the winter months and are even emitted from fluorescent light.

It is sensible to use a daily moisturiser with sunscreen filters; it can prevent premature ageing but cannot repair damage already done or reverse the process.

The Body Shop's Aloe Vera Moisturiser contains sunscreen elements from Aloe vera and almond oil. Carrot Moisture Cream is a similar good product; the inclusion of vitamin A makes the natural screening properties of carrot oil more effective.

COLLAGEN

The closely interwoven collagen fibres give the skin its youthful look, and the slow corrosion of them are major factors in the progression of ageing skin. Creams containing collagen were at one stage heralded as a great scientific breakthrough, but there is no evidence to show that collagen in creams will bind with the body's natural collagen to create younger-looking skin.

Tip: DIY tomato mask
Wash your face with a cut-up fresh tomato, rubbing it thoroughly into the skin. Leave for 5 minutes, then rinse off with clear water. Tomatoes contain an acid which peels off dead skin cells.

MALE SKIN

THROUGHOUT HISTORY, MEN HAVE PREENED AND BEAUTIFIED themselves, anointing their bodies with rich oils, heady perfumes – and tattoos and warpaints. Nero, the effeminate Roman emperor, "married" his freedman Doryphorus wearing a dress, veil and cosmetics, and another emperor, the debauched Marcus Aurelius Antoninus, made his triumphal entry into Rome in long silken robes and a tall mitre, his eyes decorated with blue and gold, his lips painted gold, and his hands and feet reddened with henna.

Rich and idle noblemen strutted like painted peacocks through royal courts right until the reign of Queen Victoria when males became sombre and dull-looking

Warning: shaving
Aerosol shaving foams have high perfume levels and aerosol propellants; they are likely to cause skin irritation.

Tip: on aftershaves
Perfumed aftershaves
sting the skin after shaving.
Use them like women use
perfume: splashed round
the neck and chest, on
elbow grooves and wrists.

Tip: for male skin
Creams based on cocoa
butter are preferable to
those with a high glycerine
content; the latter tends to
lather when applied to
whiskers.

creatures. The disdain for personal adornment, whether in dress or "beauty preparations", continued until the last quarter of the 20th century. The fact that men daily use soaps, toothpastes, shampoos, conditioners, shaving creams and after-shaves is, in male opinion, a matter of hygiene, not of cosmetics. When perfumes for men were introduced earlier this century, they appeared in the guise of "after-shaves", and the various brand names had a strong ring of masculinity.

Today, this attitude is changing rapidly, and male skin care is no longer viewed with suspicion or restricted to a splash of astringent or aftershave. With the growing interest in fitness and health, men are beginning to care what they look and feel like. Athletes and men engaged in outdoor occupations use protective skin creams, and those who want to look healthy and tanned all year round are taking to lightly tinted creams. The punk fashion has also had repercussions with the younger generation adopting colour cosmetics, bright hair dyes, eyeliners and kajal sticks.

SKIN CARE
Most men are still wary of admitting to using moisturisers even if they have un-comfortably dry skin, and male moisturising products are carefully labelled after-shave balms or soothers. Because men's skin is often oilier than women's, they do need lighter moisturisers – products like our Vitamin E Day Cream are ideal – and many of the ordinary mass-marketed women's moisturisers are perfectly adequate. Men with dry or tight skin are advised to use a moisturiser after shaving and showering, and as protection against chapping and soreness in cold, windy weather.

WASHING AND CLEANSING
The effect on the skin of washing with soap is the same for men as for women, and many men find that ordinary toilet soaps are too drying for facial use. Superfatted soaps are preferable for dry or sensitive skins, clear glycerine soaps for normal or oily skins. **Wash the face before shaving;** hot water helps to soften the beard while washing after shaving disrupts the acid mantle.

FACIAL SCRUBS
Men are as prone as women to spots, pimples and dull skin. A facial scrub is the ideal treatment and perfect for clearing up blackheads and oily patches, particularly round the nose and chin. Mix a teaspoonful of Japanese Washing Grains to a paste with a drop of water in the palm and massage it gently into the nose and chin areas; rinse off with cold water. Shaving is in itself exfoliation, leaving the skin beneath smooth and soft – a facial scrub should be taken above the beard line.

BODY

BODY CHEMISTRY

BODY CARE

HAND AND ARM CARE

LEG AND FOOT CARE

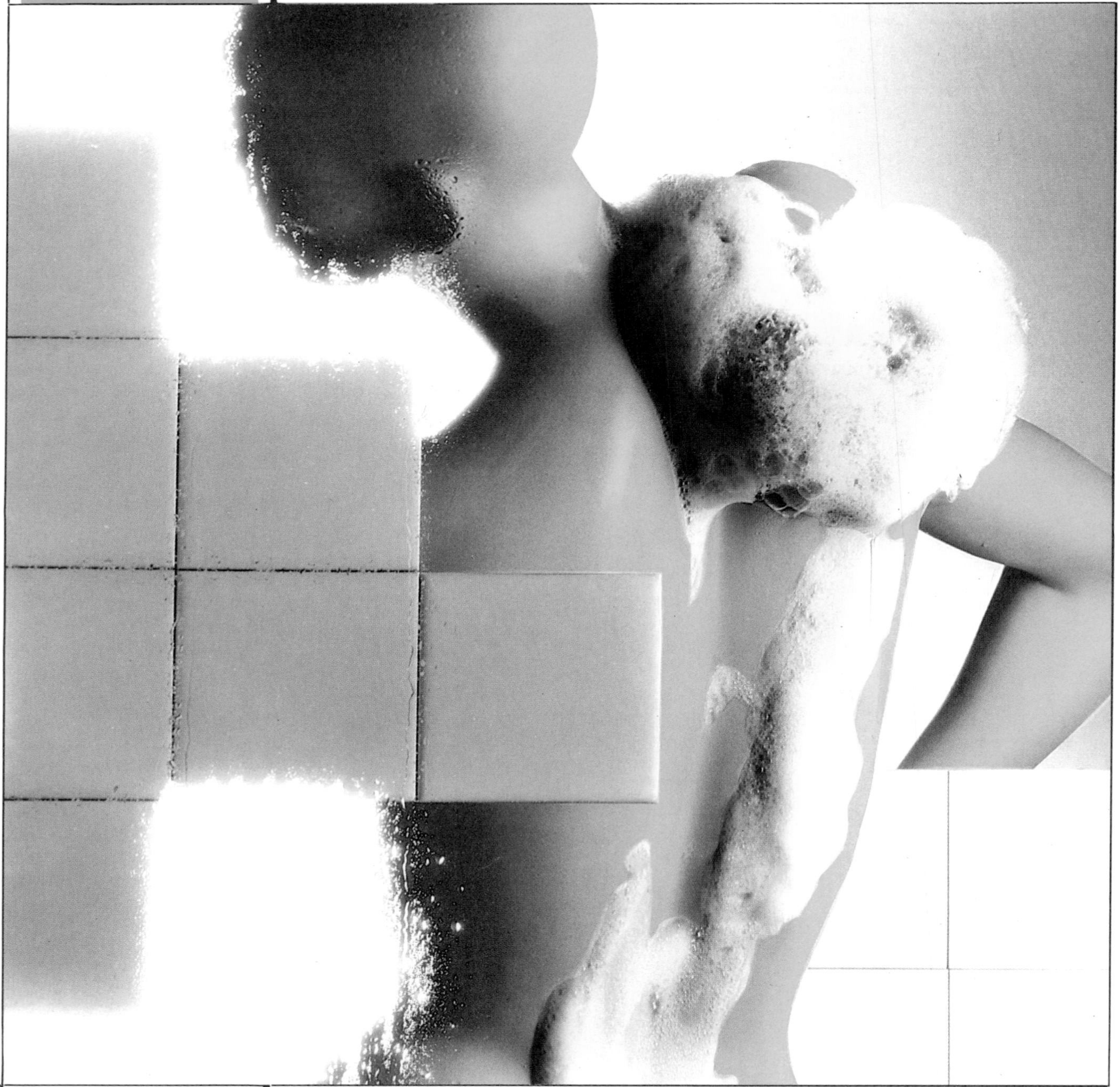

BODY CHEMITRY

THE BODY SHOP'S NAME WAS A DELIBERATE CHOICE, A STATEMENT and a reminder that skin care does not begin and end at the chin. It involves the whole body, from the tip of your toe to the top of your head, the visible as well as the invisible parts.

The body is a miraculous machine, more endurable than any invention by man, for it keeps functioning in spite of constant neglect and abuse. For most of the time we take the body for granted and only become aware of it when some part or other is damaged. Compare the body to the car, that almost indispensible machine which blocks our streets, assaults our ears and fouls the air we breathe: we wash and polish the paintwork, check meticulously the level of oil and water, choose the right grade of petrol, and take it for regular servicing. And when it no longer performs to our satisfaction, we exchange it for another model.

The most unmechanically-minded of us would admit that gleaming paintwork is of little importance if the internal parts are in poor working order. Just so with the body. We subject it to incredible maltreatment, fill it with junk food, unknown chemicals, alcohol, drugs and nicotine, contort the limbs into unnatural postures and overload the internal systems with stressful life-styles. We dehydrate our bodies in centrally-heated rooms, cleanse them, externally and internally, in chemically-treated water, swim in seas polluted with detergents and other indescribable wastes, breathe air laden with petrol fumes, chimney grime and atomic spillage. And feel amazed when the body objects and refuses to function.

MORE THAN SKIN-DEEP

It doesn't have to be like that. There is a growing interest in health and fitness, an increased awareness of ourselves and our environment, and with it opposition to the artificiality that besets life in the latter part of the 20th century. We are rediscovering that in many respects nature does know best, and we increasingly reject chemical additives or replacements, in food, cleansing and cosmetic products.

Most of us are born with the requisite number of body components, and by taking care of them all we can ensure health and looks, and stave off premature signs of advancing years. *Feeling good is looking good.*

The skin performs a number of functions; it acts as a tough protective covering for bones and muscles, nerves, blood vessels and internal organs and at the same time as a sensitive barometer for temperature, pain and other sensations. It consists of two layers, the thin outer epidermis of dead cells, and the lower and deeper layer, the dermis, made up of living, dividing cells. Embedded in the dermis and supported by bunchy twigs of collagen and flexible elastin fibres are tiny capillary blood vessels and nerve endings, as well as hair follicles, sweat and sebaceous glands.

The skin is not uniform in texture and structure; it is thinnest on the lips, thickest on the soles of the feet; hair follicles are most abundant on the scalp, absent on the

Fact: ageing gracefully
If you practise good body care from the start, ageing is a slow and gradual process: the body's biochemical activity diminishes by only 10-15% during the ages of 30 and 60.

Fact: beauty sleep
The skin regenerates itself during sleep, the body chemistry working on cell renewal, protein build-up and waste secretion.

Opposite: *Basic body care begins with cleansing, using soap or body shampoo to loosen dirt and dead cells, water to rinse off the suds, and sponge or flannel to polish the skin and to stimulate blood circulation.*

Fact: antibiotics
Every time you take an
antibiotic, it upsets the
skin's natural flora.

The skin *is the largest body
organ, enveloping bones
and muscles, nerves, blood
vessels and internal organs
with a resilient covering
which in the adult
approximates half a dozen
tea towels.*

palms of the hands; sweat glands are concentrated in the armpits, nerve-endings —
and touch sensation — in the fingertips. Skin acts as a barrier, preventing fluid and
nutrient loss from inner organs, fighting off the invasion of harmful bacteria and sun
radiation, and regulating body temperature.

The top of the skin plays host to a microflora of living bacteria. They migrate on to
the skin of the newborn baby and remain there for the rest of its life, as individual as
fingerprints, always multiplying and renewing themselves — 100 million exist in each
armpit alone. Purely beneficial to the skin in warding off potentially harmful invaders,
the microflora can become a cause of illness if it penetrates below the skin and
invades the mucuous membranes of, for example, the mouth and the vagina.

THE SKIN'S LIFE-CYCLE

The outer dead skin layer is shed continuously as cells from the dermis push their
way upwards. Millions of microscopic skin particles are sloughed off every day — a
pair of socks, for example, traps 190 milligrams of dead skin daily. It is a natural,
regenerative process, and the sloughed-off skin is removed by cleansing or caught in
clothing; if it is allowed to remain it settles as a thick layer, as on the heels, knees and
elbows, impervious to moisture and rife for cracks and bacterial invasion. The
continuous renewal and shedding of the skin, the life-cycle, takes 21-28 days.
Obviously, the shorter the cycle, the brighter and smoother the surface skin. It is
important to accelerate the renewal process by cleansing the entire body skin.

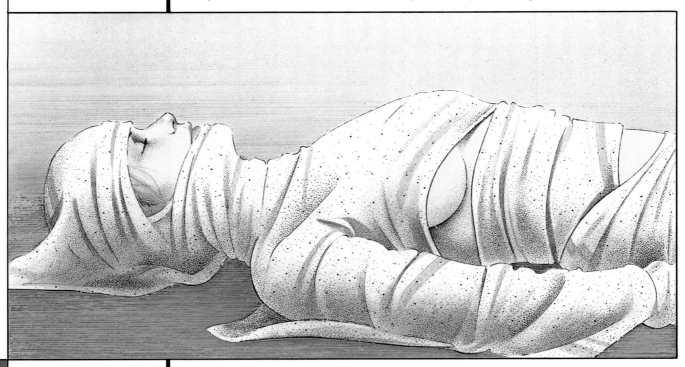

THE INNER SELF

Barring illnesses and accidents, the body structure beneath the skin – bones and muscles – and the various internal systems (nerves, respiration, circulation, digestion) function on an input-output basis. **What you get out of your body depends on what you put into it.** For healthy body growth and maintenance you need protein (vegetable and animal), starchy carbohydrates: fibre (*you don't need sugar* or chocolate), fatty acids (more for growth, less for maintenance, and poly-unsaturated rather than saturated fats), minerals, especially calcium and iron – and much less salt than you think – and vitamins. Most important are vitamins C and those of the B complex; they are soluble in water and must be replenished daily.

You need air – fresh air when you can get it – to keep the respiratory system functioning and sending vital oxygen to all parts of the body via the blood. Revive yourself, first thing in the morning, and during the day when energy is flagging, with a few breathing exercises: inhale deeply through the nose and hold the breath until you can feel the lungs emptying of stale gases; exhale *slowly*, again through the nose, and repeat several times.

All the body organs need oxygen to survive – and oxygen is transported through the blood vessels, pumped through by the constant action of the heart. It is essential that the vessels remain pliable and uncluttered; it is thought that obesity, alcohol, drugs including nicotine, and lack of exercise thicken the walls of the blood vessels and constrict the free flow of oxygen-rich blood and essential nutrients.

BODY CHEMISTRY

Fact: bacteria growth
Within 10 hours of a bath, the bacterial population on the skin has multiplied by three. No matter how hard and how long you scrub, 20% of the bacteria will be resistant to anti-bacteriacides and start new colonies.

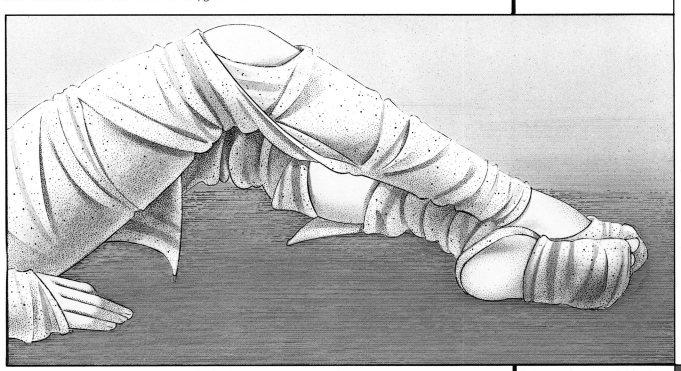

Opposite: *Soap is the
skin's best friend, foaming
with water to gentle suds
which deep-cleanse and
soothe. Translucent
glycerine soaps are
especially mild, with added
vitamin E for healthy tissue
growth.*

SLEEP – THE NATURAL RESTORER

There is a saying that the hours spent asleep before midnight count as beauty sleep; there is probably some truth in this in so far as the chances are that you are in for the healthy seven or eight hours' sleep that the average working person needs. Some people can do with less and others require more in order to function properly during the daytime. But we all need sleep, the period of rest when the brain's activities slow down, and the body's chemistry gets to work, processing the nutrients we have taken on board during the day, and healing and repairing tired or damaged tissues.

The skin in particular benefits from sleep; limbs and muscles are relaxed, the skin smooths out, erasing at least temporarily wrinkles and worry lines, and the cells can get on with their restorative work because body energy, though lower than during the day, is not diverted to anything else. Caring for your body includes listening to the signals it sends out and allowing it the necessary rest. Take a bath or shower before retiring, partly to help the muscles relax and partly to allow the skin pores to breathe; *never* go to bed without removing all face make-up and applying a moisturising night cream, such as Jojoba Night Cream or Aloe Vera Moisture Cream for normal and combination skins, Avocado Moisture Cream for oily skin, and Rich Night Cream with Vitamin E for ageing, dry and sensitive skins.

POSTURE AND EXERCISES

You do not have to be a fitness fanatic to know that regular exercise contributes to the general feeling of well-being. Exercising is rarely successful as a slimming aid on its own, but has other, equally important advantages: it improves circulation, speeds up the digestive processes, keeps muscles and limbs supple, and sweeps the cobwebs from tired brains. Try to spend at least ½ hour outdoors every day, even if it is only a brisk walk to the office – much better than hanging from a strap in an Underground train or bus. And walk upstairs instead of using the lift.

Posture is important, whether you are sitting, standing or walking. Wrong posture can lead to figure faults, especially on the back and hips, resulting in aches and sometimes permanent displacement of the spine. A well-tuned body, muscles and limbs extended to their full potentials, gives an impression of youthfulness and vitality, and prevents the sagging outline indicative of middle-age spread.

Standing straight Not like a soldier to attention, but at ease. Straighten the spine, as if an invisible cord was pulled from the top of the head, with shoulders lifted back, relaxed so that the arms pull downwards from the sockets, chest high, and head aligned with the ground. Pull in the stomach muscles to tilt the pelvis, tuck the buttocks under and keep the knees slightly bent, with the body resting on the balls of the feet. Practise standing correctly while you wait for the bus, and eventually you will do it automatically, thereby strengthening the supporting muscles.

Walking tall Progress from the standing position, back straight, shoulders back and arms relaxed, swinging naturally; use the motion muscles in the thighs, not the hips, to propel you forwards, and breathe deeply in and out.

Sitting pretty More back problems are probably due to bad sitting postures than to any other cause. Whether you are simply sitting or sitting working at a desk, the right chair is essential; it should support the spine from the base and the height adjusted so that the feet rest comfortably on the floor and the forearms from the elbows are level with the table top, forming a 90° angle.

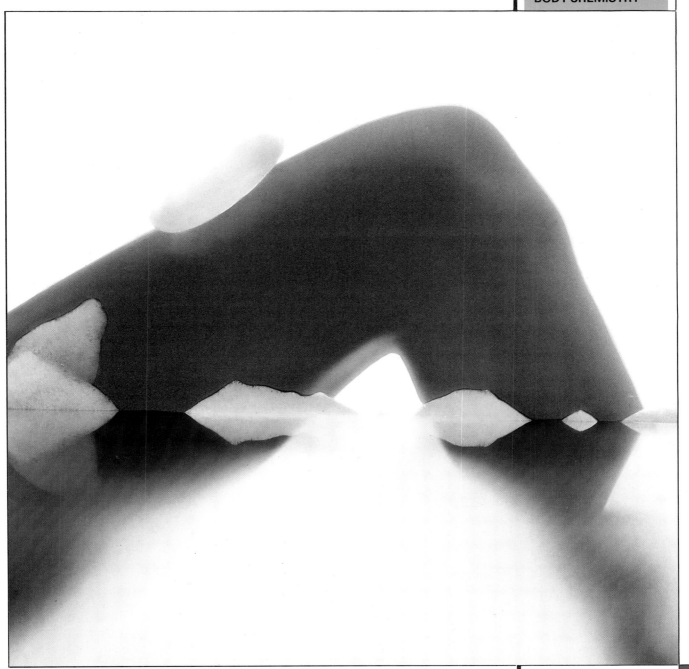

Danger: hard water
The combination of salts and minerals in hard water interacts with soap to form a residue difficult to rinse off the skin – and the bath. Rainwater, before it became polluted, was recommended for skin and hair care; today use Body Shop Herbal Bath Salts to soften hard tap water.

Tip: dry skin and water
Avoid hot baths if your skin is very dry. The natural moisturising factor in the skin is destroyed by very hot water and by prolonged soaking.

A WOMAN'S AGE

The body is constantly changing. From the moment we reach physical maturity, in the late teens, we are theoretically and inevitably on the road to degeneration. Just how quickly and obviously we progress along this path is largely up to ourselves. Proper body care, which also includes a sensible diet and regular exercise, will help us to look and feel youthful and eventually to age gracefully.

THE TEENS

This phase in a woman's life is one of immense upheaval, matched only by the point at the other end of the scale, the menopause. It is all due to tremendous hormonal activities, effecting numerous bodily and emotional changes. Feminine contours develop rapidly, and rarely in the desired proportions; emotions switch from dizzy ecstasy to utter gloom at the sight of a pimple or spot, and energy levels can plummet because of all the bodily changes.

Adequate rest is a must, and so is a proper diet. There is one enormous advantage: youth, an unappeased zest for life, a joy in experimenting and discovering. It is also the time when the foundations are laid for the later phases of the life-cycle, a time to establish a sound regimen for body care, learning to look after your hair, skin, hands and feet. **Ignore all the advertising copy and concentrate on the two basics: cleansing and protecting.** Even if you display no allergies, you can minimize the risk of allergic skin reactions in later years by choosing simply-formulated products whose ingredients are as close to source as possible.

MENSTRUATION AND WATER RETENTION

For many women, the monthly period is accompanied by unpleasant side-effects, including headaches, irritability and depression, sore breasts, muscular and abdominal pains and a feeling of bloatedness. The latter is due to water retention, and it is quite common to gain a couple of kilograms in weight prior to menstruation, and to lose them again over the first few days of the period.

You can often obtain some relief from these symptoms by reducing fluid intake and by eating frequently during the two or three days prior to menstruation. You are twice as likely to show allergic reactions just before a period. The skin may feel puffy and be unable to absorb creams properly; such symptoms often disappear over the years, during and following pregnancy and with the use of the contraceptive pill. Continuous water retention at menstruation, with attendant symptoms of pain and irritability, needs medical attention, and possibly hormone treatment.

THE PEAK YEARS

The twenties and thirties are the years when early body care really pays off, in supple limbs, healthy, shiny hair and glowing skin. Such outward attributes help to bolster self-confidence, poise and emotional tranquility. It is the time when a woman contemplates marriage, child-bearing or a career, or a mixture of these, and when life is so full that she is tempted to ignore essential body care or trust to luck that her looks will last.

They won't, and neglect now will show up the ravages within a few years. It is especially important to look after the skin and protect it against drying-out and exposure to sun; make sure it is scrupulously cleaned every night.

PREGNANCY AND STRETCH MARKS

Tremendous hormonal upheavals take place in the body during pregnancy and are reflected in the skin and the hair, often reversing from oily to dry or *vice versa*. Cleanse and moisturise for the current condition, stick to a healthy diet, with plenty of fresh fruit and vegetables, wholemeal cereal products and pulses, poultry and fish in preference to red meat. Exercise daily, especially with walking and swimming.

The skin darkens naturally during pregnancy, particularly round the nipples; dark lines may appear on the abdomen and elsewhere, and moles and freckles become more pronounced. Such discoloration is quite normal and usually disappears after the birth. However, sunbathing can make it more pronounced; be especially careful in the choice of sun preparations, or better still, stay covered up. Consult a doctor if moles and freckles appear to be growing rapidly. Varicose veins can be a major problem. Relaxin, a hormone produced during pregnancy, slows down the return supply of blood; gentle exercise can help to minimize varicose veins.

As soon as possible after the birth, begin the fight to regain your figure. Post-natal clinics usually issue diet sheets and recommend exercises aimed at restoring elasticity to the abdominal muscles. Stretch marks are common, but they can be minimized by massaging the abdomen, and the buttocks, with penetrating lubricants; the marks are more pronounced on dry skin, so start prevention as soon as pregnancy is confirmed; we recommend such natural products as Almond Oil or Cocoa-Butter Body Lotion. After the birth, regular abdominal massage with Wheatgerm Oil helps to heal the scars.

MATURITY AND AGEING

Middle-age does not happen from one day to the next; it is a gradual process in tune with a slowing-down of the body's regenerative powers and its responses to external and internal factors. A woman, who has looked after her body, can meet the challenge of the forties and fifties with equanimity and disguise the thickening waist and the slackening muscles well into her sixties.

Ageing *does* occur: the skin gradually loses its elasticity and natural moisture; the hair tends to become sparser and drier, while conversely facial hairs may increase along with a fine network of broken veins. A healthy diet, suitable exercise, correct posture and proper rest are all important. No cream or lotion can halt or reverse the passage of time, and no miracle cure can erase wrinkles or lines, but to some extent we are able to control the visible signs of the years with careful and regular grooming.

Have periodic medical check-ups, not just with the doctor, but also with the dentist and optician. Change your hairstyle; short and simple is often the most attractive, and an expert cut is a must. Steer clear of harsh chemical colourants and use less permanent waving, blow-drying and brushing.

The skin, on body and face, needs more attention than before. Add oils or water softeners to the bath, moisturise the entire body with a good oil or lotion; at night pay special attention to cleansing the face, first with cream, then with a mild soap and rinse thoroughly, avoiding very hot and very cold water. Apply a night moisturising cream, Rich Night Cream round the eyes and over throat and neck. During the day, use a good moisturiser, stick to pale tones of make-up and avoid highly coloured foundations, bright lipsticks, eyeshadows and eye liners; use a magnifying mirror when making up.

BODY CHEMISTRY

Tip: pregnancy itch
Itchy skin can be soothed with an infusion of nettle leaves steeped in hot water for 10 minutes, strained and cooled. Vaginal thrush can be alleviated, according to the National Childbirth Trust, by smoothing natural yoghourt over the vaginal area.

Warning: steroids
During pregnancy, NEVER use any kind of topical steroids to clear up skin conditions.

Fact: ageing skin
After the age of 40, the skin gets thinner which makes it all the more susceptible to environmental damage.

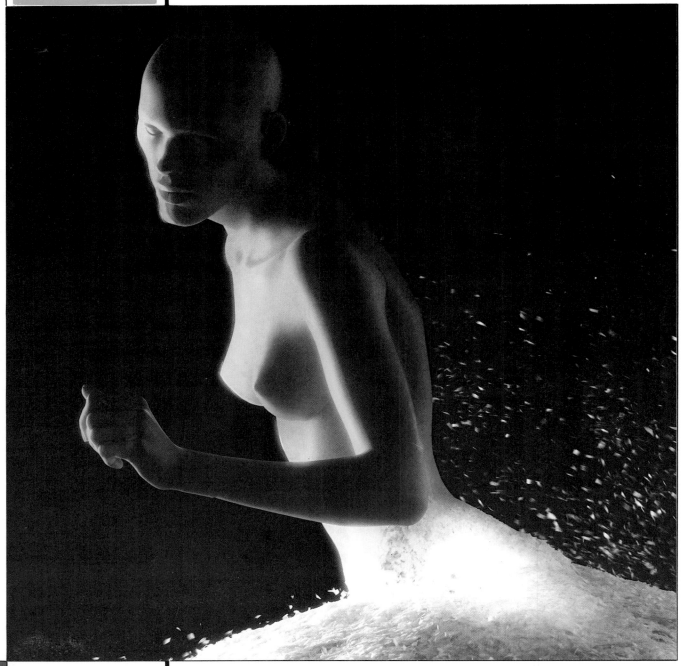

THE MENOPAUSE

About the only good thing of this phase is the relief when it is over. Some women do pass through the change of life with only minor symptoms, but for the majority the menopause is a period of dramatic changes, bodily and emotionally. Medically, the production of ova decreases and eventually stops, and with it a dimunition in the female hormone, oestrogen. The system is thrown into chaos until the body has established a new hormone balance. This process, which may last for several years, is typically accompanied by "hot flushes" which spread from the chest over neck and face, causing blushing and perspiration, sometimes strong enough to interfere with sleep. On the other hand, some women experience hardly any side-effects.

Other symptoms of the menopause include varicose veins, dry or blotchy skin, brittle nails and loss of body hair, tiredness, tears and depression, a feeling of insecurity and even suicidal notions. All these symptoms rarely occur simultaneously and do not affect all women. Hormone treatment with oestrogen, under medical guidance, can prove helpful, and a positive attitude to this temporary phase is invaluable. Today, when a women's lifespan is upwards of 80, the menopause marks merely the middle point, with several future decades spent in calmer waters.

THE MALE PHASES

These are less clearly defined though the teenage years are as turbulent for the young man as for the young woman. The body begins to assume its masculine shape, the skin to suffer from acne and spots and stubbly hair growth; and the emotions follow a steady zig-zag course. The recommendations already made for body and skin care apply equally to the young male.

The middle mature years discriminate in favour of men: greying temples and eyebrows give them distinction, the facial lines speak of decision and purpose, and middle-age spread is far more acceptable in the male than in his female contemporary. Men sometimes experience a kind of menopause, better described as a mid-life crisis in that it is emotional, not hormone linked.

BODY CARE

THE FIRST PRIORITY IS CLEANLINESS, TO RID THE SKIN OF GRIME and grease, dead cells, harmful germs and bacteria, and unpleasant body odours. Soap and water are the best cleansing agents, for skin and for clothes; underwear should ideally be changed daily, because dead skin and body odours are deposited in them.

Protection of the skin is as important as cleansing it; any soap worth its name must by necessity be degreasing and remove some of the skin's natural oil; apply a suitable body/hand lotion or cream after every bath or shower, especially on areas constricted by tight clothing.

Danger: water nymphs
You can have too many baths. Sensitive and ageing skins especially can become red and itchy from over-frequent bathing. One bath a day is sufficient; take a quick shower if you want to refresh yourself again.

Tip: bath treats
Relax tired muscles and joints in a soothing bath: dissolve 450g of Epsom salts in warm water and massage lightly with a mitt or loofah while you relax in the bath. For an invigorating bath, substitute Epsom salts with sea salts.

Opposite: *Dead cells clog the pores, encouraging spots and making the skin look dull and grey. Exfoliation at bath-time cleans and polishes the skin, stimulates circulation and enhances the feeling of well-being.*

BODY

Myth breaker: cleanliness
Many Victorian mothers sewed their children into their underwear, sometimes smeared with goose fat, at the beginning of winter and did not unpick it until spring. It kept the cold and chills out, but neither child nor vest were ever washed until spring. The practice continued well into the 20th century.

Fact: public baths
Only recently has bathing become a private affair. Roman baths were communal and mixed, Norman families bathed together with their guests, and at Bath in the 17th century, mixed and nude bathing was visible from the street. Until the advent of running water, bathing was done in a tub in front of the fire, with servants to fetch and carry water.

SOAKING IN THE TUB

According to a report on bathing habits in Britain, 60% of all women have a daily bath, compared with 45% of men. Housewives and students come out top, averaging three and a half baths a week, students soaking for longer than anyone else, on average 32 minutes compared with 29 minutes for teenagers, 26 minutes for men and 24 minutes for women. Wednesday is the favourite bath day, with almost half the adult population performing their ablutions.

The shower is less popular in Britain than in other Western countries, despite its obvious advantages: it is less time-consuming and uses much less water than the bath; the water temperature is more constant, and rinsing is more effective than lying in a bath replete with soapy scum and flakes of skin. On the other hand, a good soak in the tub is an opportunity for relaxing and unwinding, for letting facial and hair treatments get to work and for toning the skin with a massage mitt.

THE HISTORY OF BATHING

We consider our standards of hygiene to be high, and compared to the Middle Ages they probably are; viewed on the background of the Ancient World they are almost deplorable! Archaeological digs in Mesopotamia, the cradle of Western civilization, have unearthed luxurious bathrooms dating from about 3000 BC and complete with running hot and cold water and bath tubs similar to those of today.

The Ancient Greeks, who idolized the human body, built baths as adjuncts to the gymnasia where form and muscles were perfected. The Romans had their bath houses with hot sweat rooms, where the senators would cleanse their bodies with oil, and cooling rooms or *frigidaria*, where they would socialize and gossip for hours. For the Mohammedans, daily purification in hot water was an intrinsic part of religious life, and instrumental in keeping contagious diseases at bay. The Hindus bathed daily in perfumed waters, as a preliminary to love-making.

In the cold northern Europe, bathing was probably practised only during the summer months; the stench so offended the Roman invaders in the first century that they built elaborate bath-houses wherever they settled, including the famous Aquae Sulis at Bath, renowned for its warm mineral springs. When the Romans departed in the fourth century, the native population returned to their slovenly habits. Returning Crusaders attempted to establish Turkish baths, but they quickly degenerated into houses of ill repute and infection.

Medieval monks bathed, in cold water as a penitence, and so did the noblemen on whom were conferred the knighthood of the Order of the Bath, instituted in 1603, though in this instance the bath had the purely symbolic significance of purity. By Tudor times the washing process had accelerated to a monthly bath, for the aristocracy at least, but dirt and body odours were still mainly disguised with powders and perfumes, the puritanical antics of Cromwell notwithstanding.

Hard on the heels of the Renaissance, the revival of classical ideas, came a new notion of personal cleanliness, and the rich took to installing bathrooms on a sumptuous scale. Under the influence of Beau Brummel (1778-1840), the leader of fashionable society of the day, the Prince Regent, later George IV, installed a royal bathroom at the Brighton Pavilion where the rich young men soaked for hours in baths of hot water and milk. Few people, even among the rich, could afford such extravagances, and while baths were the order of the day at great public schools, they were of the cold variety, supposedly in order to develop manliness in the face of adversity and to quell the ardours of puberty. Wellington, to the end of his life, insisted on a daily cold bath, unlike Napoleon who had his tub of hot water and perhaps for that reason met his Waterloo!

Affluent Victorians were great believers in cleanliness; Mrs Beaton advocated a warm bath, of short duration, twice a week in winter, every other day in summer for those in robust health, and believed in cold baths as an aid to promoting and preserving vigour! At the turn of this century, few houses were built with bathrooms, and water still had to be heated on the kitchen range and carried to the bath tub. It is only since the Second World War that piped hot water has become commonplace and the daily bath regarded as routine, not a luxury.

THE SLIPPERY STORY OF SOAP

Primitive man probably used the sandy and abrasive grains of sea and river shores to cleanse the body, progressing to a mixture of wood ashes and animal fat. Later he discovered the cleansing values of saponin, a chemical substance contained in the leaves, roots and barks of many plants, including the Egyptian and Spanish soap-root, the soap-bark from Chili, and our native soapwort. Natural saponin is used as an ingredient in Body Shop shampoos.

The Phoenicians are credited with the development of soap manufacture. The great seafarers traded their luxury goods along the Mediterranean countries in the

BODY CARE

Fact: bath milk
Mary Queen of Scots had a stone bath-house built outside the walls of Holyrood Palace at Edinburgh, where she bathed in asses' milk or wine. Another queen, Nero's Poppeia, always travelled with a train of asses to provide milk for her daily bath.

BODY CARE AT A GLANCE					
	DRY SKIN	**SENSITIVE SKIN**	**ACNE-PRONE SKIN**	**AGEING SKIN**	**NORMAL SKIN**
BATHING	Daily	Daily	Daily	Daily	Daily
SOAP	Jojoba Oil	Goat's Milk with Honey Lily Milk	Vitamin E Glycerine with Almond	Orchid Oil	Glycerine Fruit
BATH ACCESSORIES	Bath Oil	Herb Body Shampoo	Herbal Bath Tablets	Raspberry Ripple Bath Oil	Bath Salts/Oils
TALCUM POWDER		Daily		Daily	Daily
DEODORANT	Daily	Daily	Daily	Daily	Daily
EXFOLIATION	Sponge/shaving brush	Sponge	Loofah	Loofah mitt	Loofah/sisal mitt
SPECIAL TREATS	Rich Massage Lotion Neroli Aromatherapy Oil	Herb Body Shampoo Chamomile Aromatherapy Oil	Bath Oil Powder	Rose Absolute Aromatherapy Oil	Orange Cream Bath Oil

Fact: on ablutions
The Japanese really practise cleanliness, washing in one bath and relaxing in another bath of clean water. Europeans cheerfully wallow in their own dirty ablutions. If this turns you off, take a shower; it uses much less water, is more invigorating and better for dry skin.

5th century BC, and the art of soap-making eventually spread throughout Gaul. The Celts introduced soap to Iron-Age Britain when they invaded from across the Channel, and commercial enterprises were established in Spain, France and Italy in the early centuries of the Christian era.

TOILET SOAPS

Throughout the Middle Ages, soaps were used almost exclusively for the washing of clothes. Bodies, when they were washed at all, were cleansed with toilet waters and heavily perfumed to disguise the smell of dirt. Monopolies by zealous soap guilds, high taxation and inflated prices ensured that fine toilet soap was a luxury only the rich could afford. Napoleon is said to have paid exorbitant prices for the bars of Brown Windsor soap he favoured, and when William Gladstone, as Chancellor of the Exchequer, finally abolished the soap tax in 1853, he did so reluctantly, labelling soap as "injurious to the comfort and health of the people".

Cheap laundry and toilet soap remained pretty much the same. It came in long bars and was cut into chunks of the desired size by the shopkeepers. In 1884 William Hesketh Lever had the bright idea of marketing soap in ready-cut bars, each individually stamped with his brand name "Sunlight". It was a smelly affair, quickly turning rancid on exposure to air, and Lever's next step along the commercial road was to wrap each bar separately in paper and to add citronella as a perfume to toilet soaps.

Bath gels, *salts and crystals (far right) soften hard tap water, but more importantly help to cleanse and moisturise the skin. The scent is an extra bonus, and the luxurious feeling of relaxation is beneficial for body and mind.*

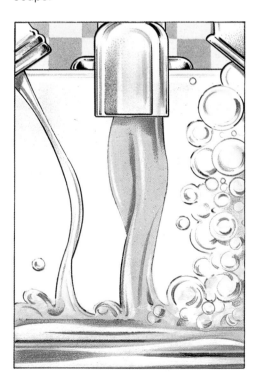

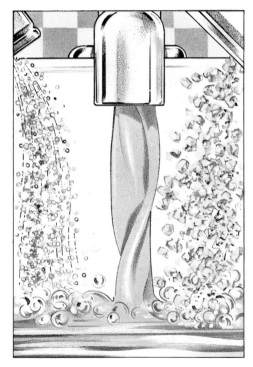

MODERN SOAPS

Today, soaps are formulated to suit different skin types, mass-produced or hand-made, at corresponding prices. **Soap and water remain the most efficient ingredients for cleansing,** and adverse reactions to soap are usually due to improper rinsing, too harsh a formulation on sensitive skin, and lack of a moisturiser.

For dry skin, we recommend a superfatted soap like our Jojoba Oil Soap and for sensitive skins, including children's, gentle Goat's Milk with Honey Soap. Connoisseurs of soap swear by transparent glycerine soaps, in colours corresponding to their fragrances, such as Green Apple, Fresh Lemon, Mandarin and Apricot; they are especially mild, less alkaline than other soaps and while they produce less lather, they rinse off more easily. Body Shop's glycerine tablets also include Vitamin E Soap and Lily Milk Soap, both recommended for sensitive skins, and Glycerine with Almond Soap for acne-prone skins; the latter also benefit from Oatmeal Soap which soothes skin irritations and rashes.

BATH ACCESSORIES

Whether you use a flannel or a sponge for soaping and rinsing is a matter for personal preference, though flannels tend more quickly than sponges to become slimy when wet, hard and abrasive when dry, from unrinsed soap deposits.

Natural sponges are harvested from the Mediterranean sea-bed; they are the fossilized skeletons of complex marine organisms (until the 18th century they were

Fact: Sunlight soap
A crafty salesman once painted "Sunlight Soap" down the main street of Port Elizabeth, South Africa, during the dead of night. The next morning he sold the irate mayor a crate of soap with which to remove the paint.

Warning: dangerous soaps
Use medicated soap only if it has been prescribed by your doctor. On acne'd or problem skins, use Body Shop Oatmeal or Glycerine with Almond Soap.

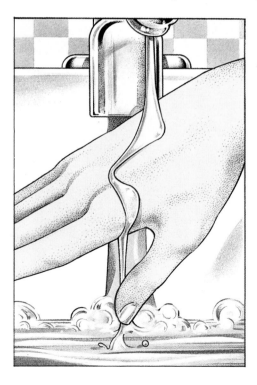
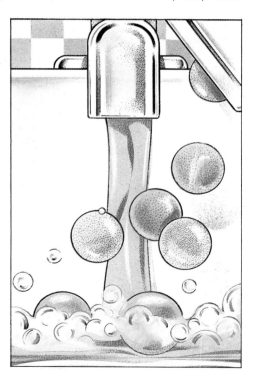

Bath oil *(far left) can be added to a hot running bath or massaged into the skin after a shower. Bubbles cleanse and soothe, veiling the skin with a delicious fragrance of perfume oils.*

Fact: spongers and soaks
The Romans soaked sea sponges in water and used them as drinking vessels; sponges also did duty as paint brushes, helmet paddings and, embedded on sticks, as washable lavatory paper. Centuries later, pulverized and burnt sponges were prescribed for gout.

Fact: smelly baths
According to a Mintel report, bubble baths, gels and oils are increasing in popularity; 35% of women use them compared with 23% who use bath salts or cubes. Bubble baths, gels and oils are favourite among the 20-24 youngsters, bath salts and cubes in the 55-64 age group.

Overleaf *"Skin care does not begin and end at the chin. It involves the whole body, from the tip of your toe to the top of your head."*

thought to be of vegetable origin or — more popularly — solidified sea foam). In composition, they are sieve-like and porous, oxygen and tiny plant and marine life washing into them with the sea water which leaves through the larger channels. Few predators attack them; tiny marine snails may nibble away at the porous masses, but the wounds heal almost as fast as they appear. They reproduce by various means of non-sexual activities, such as budding and spores which eventually form new sponges, though it takes up to five years for a sponge to reach the size of a football. They have an amazing survival capacity, being able to reform even if ground up, and tiny pieces from a living sponge culture will attach themselves and grow in suitable warm resting places.

BATH ADDITIVES

Oils or foam, gels, bubbles or beads, salt or crystals are added to the bath to cleanse or moisturise the skin or to soften the water. The scent is an additional bonus, creating an atmosphere of luxury and leaving the skin pleasantly fragrant. Always add oil, foam or salt to the bath while the hot water is gushing out, and never use more than the recommended amount; excessive doses may irritate sensitive skins. Some bath oils can be used in place of soap, such as our Foaming Bath Oil with Rose, Musk or Herb fragrance, Strawberry Body Shampoo containing a soapless cleanser, sea salt and strawberry perfume, or Herb Body Shampoo/Shower Gel, a mild soap substitute scented with alpine herbs and suitable for the most sensitive skin.

AFTER-BATH TREATMENTS

Following the bath or shower, dry the skin, thoroughly between the toes and in all creases and folds, and *apply a moisturiser while the body is still slightly damp* when the skin will best absorb oils and creams. On a daily basis, massage Cocoa-Butter Hand and Body Lotion lightly over the whole body, giving special attention to the legs which always tend to be dry because of fewer sebaceous glands; it suits all skin types and is especially beneficial to dry and sore skin, cocoa butter softening it, chamomile and marigold oils calming and soothing red and inflamed skin, and extract of myrrh oil stimulating nail growth.

As special treats, massage or spray the body with a scented Bath Oil, Raspberry Ripple Bath Oil, aromatherapy oils or our unscented Body Massage Oil which can be used as it is or scented with a few drops of one of the Perfume Oils; they are concentrates, contain no alcohol and come in a wide variety of fragrances.

Talcum powder appears to have lost its popularity, in spite of its many advantages. It helps to complete the drying process, enhances body fragrance (Body Shop's Italian talcum powders are scented with Tea Rose or Samarkand) and cools prickly heat. It prevents chafing from tight clothes and shoes and is ideal for absorbing moisture gathering beneath the breasts.

PERSPIRATION AND PERSONAL HYGIENE

The skin is constantly covered by a thin film of moisture caused by natural and essential perspiration. More than 2 million sweat glands labour to keep the body cool and the skin protected from ultraviolet light; even on a chilly day, the normal adult excretes around 1 litre of perspiration. Obesity, strenuous exercise and excessive intake of alcohol and spicy food all contribute to excessive perspiration.

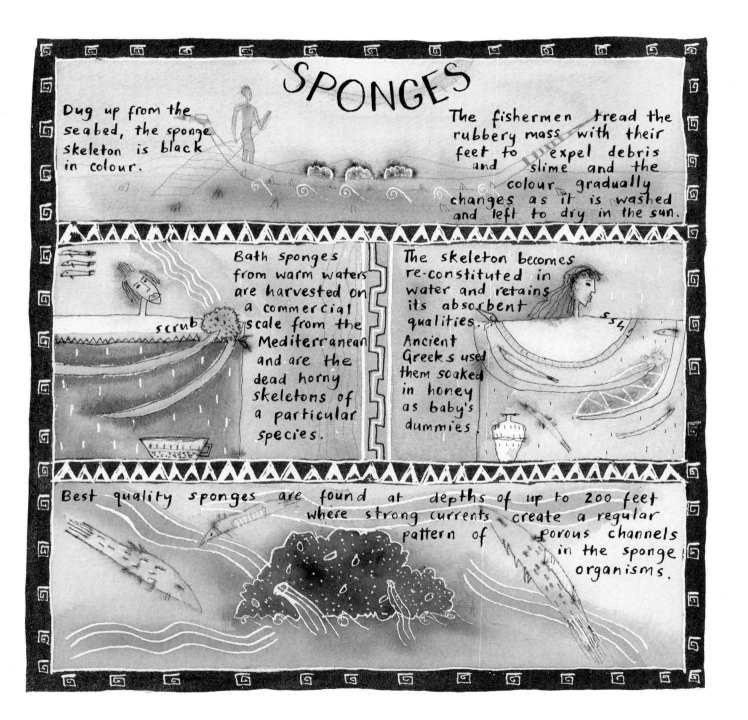

SPONGES

Dug up from the seabed, the sponge skeleton is black in colour.

The fishermen tread the rubbery mass with their feet to expel debris and slime and the colour gradually changes as it is washed and left to dry in the sun.

Bath sponges from warm waters are harvested on a commercial scale from the Mediterranean and are the dead horny skeletons of a particular species.

scrub

The skeleton becomes re-constituted in water and retains its absorbent qualities. Ancient Greeks used them soaked in honey as baby's dummies.

Best quality sponges are found at depths of up to 200 feet where strong currents create a regular pattern of porous channels in the sponge organisms.

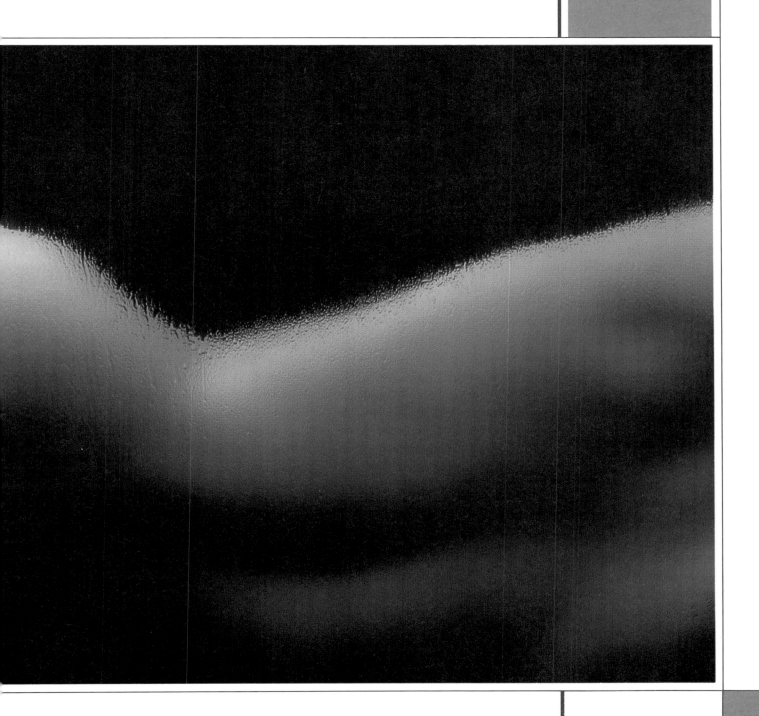

ELDERFLOWERS

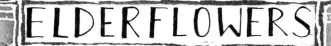

Elderflowers are used in their fresh state but, as the flowering season lasts for only three weeks they are also salted and stored. The pickled flowers are used to make Elderflower water.

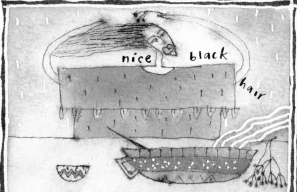

nice black hair

American Indians use elder leaves and flowers in an anti-septic wash for skin diseases and the berries to dye their hair black.

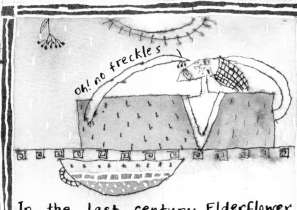

oh! no freckles

In the last century Elderflower water was used for clearing the complexion of freckles and sunburn. Its use after sea bathing was also recommended.

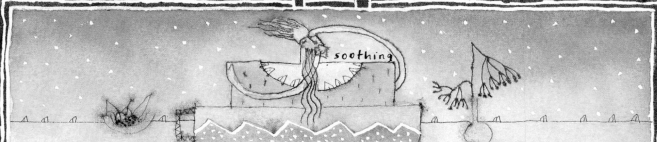

soothing

Elderflower water is an official preparation of the British Pharmacopaeia and is used mainly in eye and skin lotions.

Two types of sweat glands occur: the eccrine glands which are found throughout the body and function as heat regulators, secreting colourless and odourless water; and the apocrine glands which are clustered chiefly in the armpits and between the legs. They do not begin to function until puberty and slow down with age which is why young children and old people are rarely troubled by B.O. As well as being triggered by heat, the apocrine glands also react to emotional stress and tension and secrete a milky liquid, odourless at first but through the action of the skin's bacteria decomposing and releasing the typical ammonia-like smell.

Cleanliness, with soap and water and freshly laundered clothes daily, is the first line of defence against body odours, but because the sweat glands operate continuously it is insufficient in itself. Perspiration begins to smell after 6 hours and is strong enough to stain clothes permanently after 24 hours.

Perspiration and its treatment apply equally to men and women, though the odour-releasing apocrine glands are more numerous in females who therefore are more prone to B.O. During increased hormonal activity, such as adolescence, menstruation and pregnancy, these glands also secrete more sweat.

DEODORANTS AND ANTI-PERSPIRANTS

The two perform different functions; deodorants remove the smell - and, if perfumed, mask body odour – while anti-perspirants incorporate chemicals to check and inhibit bacterial action. In many products, the two functions are combined; the choice is vast and ranges from powders, creams, lotions and gel sticks to sprays and roll-ons. Formulations vary, and some people may experience adverse reactions, including skin irritations, from one product and none from another; often perfume acts as an irritant, in which case choose a non-perfumed preparation.

Before using a deodorant and/or anti-perspirant make sure that the skin is free of hairs, which trap bacteria, and allow 12-24 hours after depilation before using the preparation. Apply it to dry skin and give it time to dry before dressing.

EXFOLIATION

The most dramatic improvement of the skin's surface texture is through the physical removal of dead cells. We firmly believe that **exfoliation is the most effective way of creating "the optical illusion" whereby the skin looks younger.** A good scrub with a face flannel, sponge, washing grains, loofah or sisal mitt really improves the look and feel of the skin because it speeds up the cell renewal cycle.

Recent studies justify exfoliation as part of skin care. It removes surface oil, dirt and dead cells which clog up the pores and lead to spots, and loosen the blockages so that spots already formed will clear up more quickly. Exfoliation also improves flaking and red areas caused by age or sun damage; it is used to treat psoriasis and other skin conditions and can help to repair the tissues of superficial scars.

SKIN ALLERGIES

The skin on the body is less sensitive than that on the face and can generally tolerate ordinary soaps. However, the complexities of our environment, polluted by all kinds of chemicals, increasingly lead to allergies. No ingredient can be guaranteed to exclude sensitive reactions though natural ingredients have a better record than chemical compounds. At the same time, allergies are highly individual, and a product

Danger: micro killers
The outbreak of thrush in the 1960s and 1970s was largely due to harsh vaginal deodorants which disrupted the skin's microflora.

Tip: soda baths
The skin takes on an astonishing slip after a soda bath. Marvellous for itching skin, for relief from vaginitis and for children allergic to bubble baths. Pour a small tub of bicarbonate of soda into the bath and relax. You can perfume the soda with an aromatic oil: dip the tip of a cotton bud in the oil and place it in the soda, making a figure of eight to distribute the oil evenly. Cover it with the lid, shake the container and leave overnight. The soda will take on the aroma and perfume the bath.

Exfoliation tools *like natural sponges (right) and soft shaving brushes (far right) are ideal for sensitive skin areas; on back and shoulders use a loofah.*

which suits one person admirably may bring another out in a rash. The symptoms include redness, swelling, heat and pain, accompanied by itching, dry and flaky skin. Even when an allergy has been located, treated or eliminated, the skin will remain hypersensitive to other products until it has calmed down. Never use antiseptic creams on a skin in the process of recovering.

An allergy is rarely caused by a so-called bad product; it merely happens to react adversely in a few cases (if the reactions were universal, the product would obviously be withdrawn from the market). Surveys carried out in the United States have found that talcum powders and soaps carry the least risk of allergic reactions, while skin bleaches, depilatories and deodorants come top of the list.

FLOWER WATERS

Extracts from flowers and fruits are recommended for sensitive skins in place of perfumes. Many have soothing and mildly astringent properties. The Body Shop Elderflower Water is a cooling freshener, recommended as a facial tonic and for skins recovering from allergic reactions to cosmetic products. The heavily scented elder-flowers contain traces of a volatile oil used for centuries in cosmetic and medicinal preparations; this oil probably gave rise to the old Anglo Saxon name for elder, *Ellaern*, meaning to fire or kindle. The botanical name, *Sambucus*, comes from the ancient Greek word for a stringed musical instrument, sambuke, said to have been made from the wood of the elder tree.

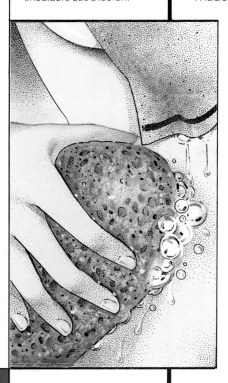

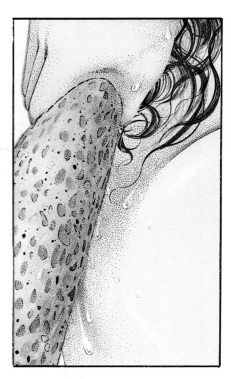

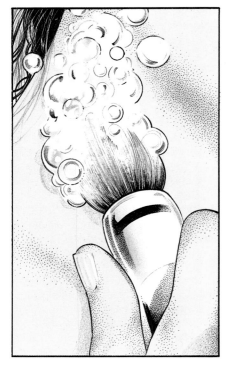

THE NECK DOWN

Facial skin care, including cleansing, toning and moisturising, should extend over the throat and neck where lines and wrinkles show up early, partly because of neglect and partly because this area contains few sebaceous glands. The so-called necklace-lines, which eventually deepen to a couple of sharply etched circles, often begin to form in the twenties unless precautions are taken. Every night, apply a rich night cream or Body Shop Neck Gel, massaging it in with the knuckles.

Dry, grey and dingy skin on neck and throat benefits greatly from exfoliation: scrub briskly with a face flannel or soft shaving brush, using a mild facial toilet soap or an Elizabethan Wash-Ball (with rose, cedarwood or spice oils); rinse thoroughly with tepid water and pat dry before massaging moisturiser into the throat.

Double chins are not necessarily caused by obesity; bad posture is equally at fault. When sitting, try not to slump and practise a few simple exercises: purse the lips and at the same time rotate the head as if your eyes were following a moving insect. You can also ease tension in the neck by letting the head drop slowly forward, then rotating it along the right shoulder and along the back, letting it drop backwards and then moving it upright; repeat along the left shoulder. More often than not you will hear a grinding, crackling noise; this is caused by calcium deposits which will gradually disperse with daily neck exercises. The age-old recipe of walking with a book balanced on top of the head encourages good posture.

BACK AND SHOULDERS

For the greater part of the year these are given only perfunctory treatment; blemishes are hidden from ourselves and onlookers until the first heatwave. Good posture and exercises to keep the spine supple and the shoulders flexible help to preserve a youthful appearance; they can also help to check the spread of "spare tyre" along the bra line although these bulges are more likely caused by overweight.

Spots are common after a winter spent in woollies and need concerted treatment before they develop into acne. In many cases, daily exfoliation with a loofah or stiff back brush is sufficient to deal with dry, flaking skin and superficial spots. If necessary, follow up with surgical spirit dabbed over particularly bad areas. Persistent spots may need treatment at dermatological clinics.

It can be difficult to massage your own back, but unless there is a friendly soul to give you a helping hand, persevere on your own and remember that the movements help to exercise back and shoulder muscles. For rough and dry skin, try a salt and oil rub, applied with a loofah or sisal mitt: dip the mitt first in warm olive or body oil, then into coarse sea salt and rub vigorously over the back and shoulders. Rinse thoroughly, rub dry and smooth in moisturising cream or lotion.

Many skins react to synthetic materials; wear cotton or silk next to the skin, loose rather than tight so that perspiration can evaporate naturally. Remember to cover the thin skin on the shoulders with adequate sunscreen protection.

BUST OR NOT

Few women are satisfied with their breasts, seeing them either as too small or too large, too pointed or too floppy. Bosoms are highly individual, differing from woman to woman, the shape and size being largely determined by inherited genes and hormone levels. Breasts contain no muscles but consist of glands, fat and fibrous

Tip: neck discoloration
Those dull, greyish lines on neck and throat can be bleached by smoothing natural yoghourt or buttermilk over the cleansed skin and leaving it for at least half an hour. Rinse off with lukewarm water.

Tip: spotty back
Dab stubborn spots, after exfoliation, with surgical spirit or an antiseptic lotion, then apply a pack: mix Fuller's earth, witchhazel or baker's yeast to a paste with facial cleansing milk. Smooth over spotty areas, leave for 20 minutes or until the pack has dried hard; rinse off with warm water.

Tip: breast press-ups
Under a hot shower, massage the breasts with strong, firm strokes, pressing upwards from beneath the breasts, over the nipples and up to the chin.

Danger: hormone creams
Hormone treatment to enlarge the bust ceases to be effective as soon as treatment is stopped. It can also interfere with the body's normal hormone balance and produce serious side-effects.

tissues supported by two large muscles, the pectorals, which extend, behind the bust, from neck to waist. Improvements in bust shape and size therefore relate to strengthening the supporting muscles and keeping the fibrous tissues supple.

Bust size is a question of proportions; if the measurement of the bust is roughly the same as the hip measurement and about 25-30cm more than that of the waist, the proportions are considered well-balanced. Shape is a different matter, and can generally be altered by simple means; a well-fitting bra which lifts and supports, without restricting circulation, flattening the nipples or pinching in the armpits, is often sufficient, and proper posture can work wonders. If you sit slumped or walk with hunched shoulders, the breasts will eventually sag.

FIRMING EXERCISES

Large breasts due to obvious obesity benefit from a reducing diet, geared to a slow but steady weight loss rather than a crash slimming course which can leave you with smaller but sagging breasts. After any appreciable weight loss or simply to tone the bosom, try to establish a daily routine, before a bath or shower, of simple exercises:

1. Stand erect, feet slightly apart, and stretch out the arms level with the shoulders; sketch large circles with the arms, first in one direction, then the other.

2. Still standing, swing the arms in front, palms downwards, then push them back as far as they will go, towards the back. Good for firming the sides of the breasts.

3. Stand, or kneel upright, with arms extended above the head; bring them slowly together and hold for a few seconds. Helps to firm the base of the bust.

Gentle massage, ideally with an aromatherapy oil of your choice, is also helpful for toning and firming the muscles and for smoothing the skin. Apply a few drops of warm oil, after a bath when the skin is warm and slightly moist, and massage with fingers and palms, in small circular movements inwards from the outer sides of each breast, and upwards from below the bust right up to the neck.

No creams or machines can enlarge the breasts, and any advertising claims to that effect operate under false, often dangerous premises. Hormonal massage creams can penetrate the skin and upset the body's hormone and glandular balance. Electrical gadgets can injure the tissues and spread undetected cancer tumours. Cosmetic surgery is possible though not to be recommended.

BREAST CANCER

One in every fifteen women is likely to develop breast cancer, more commonly after the age of 40, but detected early enough treatment is generally successful. **Not all breast lumps are malignant,** and up to 80% show up as benign during biopsy; what is dangerous is delay in reporting to your doctor any disturbing symptoms.

Get into the habit of examining the breasts every month, after the menstruation period, and seek immediate medical help if any of the following symptoms occur:

1. Discharge or bleeding from the nipples.
2. Discoloration, sinking or rising of the nipples.
3. Dimpling of the skin or marked changes in the shape.
4. A lump in the armpit or breast.

Stand naked in front of the mirror, raise the arms above the head and look carefully for depressions or changes in the shape of the breasts, overall and in one compared with the other.

Lie down flat on your back; place a pillow under the left shoulder and use the fingers of the right hand to examine the left breast: press with the flat of the fingers over the tissues extending into the armpit, where most lumps originate, then move to the upper, outer quarter of the breast before feeling the lower outer quarter, from the edge to the centre near the nipple. Examine the inner, upper half of the breast, pressing it against the rib cage and moving the fingers from the chestbone towards the centre of the breast. Feel over the nipple area, then move to the lower half. Move the pillow under the right shoulder and examine the right breast in the same way.

HIPS AND BUTTOCKS

Exercising and dieting to improve the waist also benefit the hips. Most of us lead a sedentary life; we sit in the same position for many hours, thereby restricting circulation and developing sagging muscles in hips and buttocks which spread to the typical pear shape. Whether you call this spread of tissues cellulite or flab, only exercise and massage can help to correct it. The Body Shop Body Buddy, used with a body shampoo, stimulates circulation, and you can follow up with an aromatherapy oil and a loofah mitt, massaging the flesh with upwards movements.

The buttocks often develop dry and pimply skin, probably due to friction from tight clothes or reaction to synthetic materials. Always wear cotton next to the skin and exfoliate it thoroughly with a good scrub during bathing and showering. Protect the skin with Cocoa-Butter Hand and Body Lotion, and in hot weather dust with talcum.

BODY CARE

Fact: Mum's the word
The first commercial deodorant appeared in 1890. It was a zinc oxide cream, named Mum.

Hard skin *succumbs to vigorous rubbing with coarse salt and water (far left) or pumice stone (left). Fine soft hairs can be removed with a razor: for overall, longer-lasting treatment use a leg wax.*

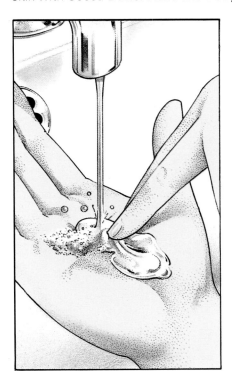

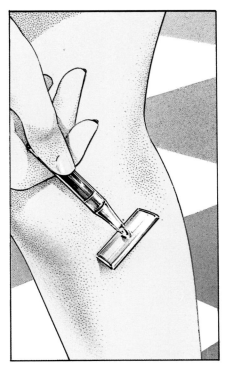

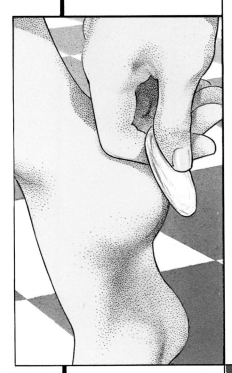

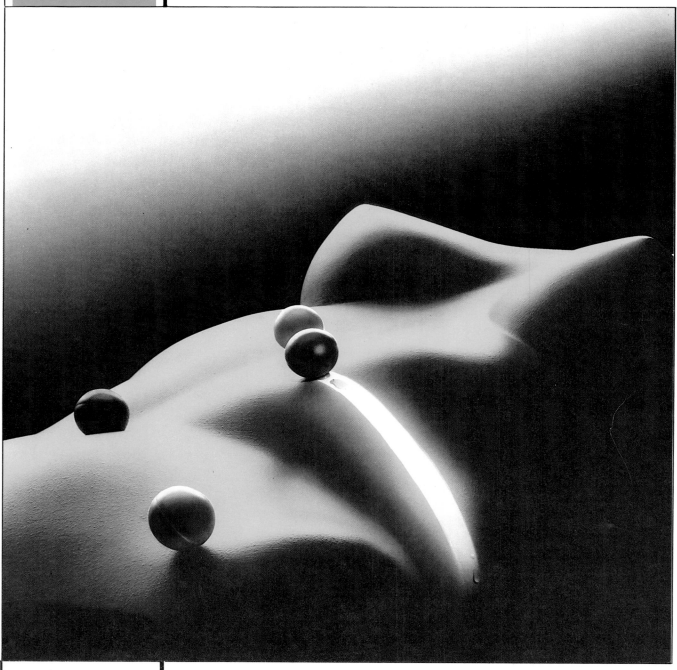

HAND AND ARM CARE

FOR MOST OF THE YEAR WE LEAVE THE ARMS TO THEIR OWN devices and only become aware of their dull, flabby appearance when we don sleeveless shirts and dresses. There is not much you can do about skinny arms, without upholstering other parts of the body, but flab is a different matter, and it gets worse with age. The sagging look of the upper arms is not necessarily related to overweight, but to lack of muscle tone.

Exercises are the only way to reduce the cellulite accumulations, and massage oils and lotions to improve the skin's elasticity. The exercises recommended for toning up the pectoral muscles behind the bust will also affect the upper arms, and you can improve circulation with the following daily routine: stand, feet a little apart, with arms stretched out in front, at shoulder level; swing them backwards, trying to make the fingertips touch at the back. Or try weightlifting: hold a heavy book in one hand, raise the arm straight above the head and bring the book to touch the back of the opposite shoulder; repeat with the other hand.

Regular exfoliation with a loofah mitt or friction glove also improves circulation and rids the skin of dead, clogging cells; on the upper arms in particular, the skin is often pimply in winter, from constant contact with rough materials. After exfoliation, massage Cocoa-Butter Hand and Body Lotion into the skin, moving from the wrists upwards, with firm strokes. In summer, protect the arms — and shoulders — with a sunscreen preparation appropriate to your skin type.

ELBOWS

These are possibly the most neglected parts of the body; we rarely catch sight of them ourselves, but to the onlooker our elbows speak eloquently of age and neglect. The thin skin quickly becomes rough and wrinkled, and because we frequently rest them on a hard table-top, grains of dirt become embedded in the wrinkles, settling to flakes and eventually to callouses.

Scrub the elbows daily with a soapy pumice stone or bristly brush until all ingrained dirt has disappeared, then bleach the reddened skin with lemon juice and massage with a good moisturiser. If you must sit with elbows resting on the desk, cup them in two squeezed-out lemon halves to soften and bleach the skin.

HANDS

Our hands reveal more about us than we realize; they are constantly on view yet we neglect them more consistently than any other feature. They are exposed to the ravages of sun and wind, cold and heat, and we immerse them in detergents, chemicals, oil and polishes. Hands reveal our physical condition to the medical eye, our character and tensions to the trained psychologist, and to the onlooker they betray our age. Faced with an important date, we become aware of our red, rough and wrinkled hands, but long-term neglect cannot be remedied overnight.

Fact: hands and age
It has been said that a woman's age shows most clearly in elbows and hands. Austrian women used to sleep with the hands tied above their heads, causing the blood to drain downwards and supposedly making the veins smaller, and the hands more attractive.

Tip: tennis elbows
Wear an elasticated support to minimize wear and fatigue and to control swelling and pain.

Opposite: *Bath oil beads contain highly concentrated oils which leave the skin smooth and supple. Leave one bead to dissolve in the bath and choose from such fragrances as lemon, apple, strawberry or rose.*

Tip: treats for hands
Cleanse garden-soiled hands by dipping them in warm oil, then rub with coarse salt and rinse off.

Keep a small bowl of bran, in which to dip hands, near the sink or washbasin; rub thoroughly to cleanse them, and rinse off.

Soap dried-out hands for half an hour in warm Sweet Almond Oil; great for nails, too.

Myth breaker: detergents
No dishwashing liquid, irrespective of advertising claims, can be "good for your hands". Any detergent effective enough to degrease crockery must also degrease the skin. Wear rubber gloves when washing up and keep a jar of hand cream by the sink.

Opposite: Massage mitts, made from sisal or loofah, are ideal for reaching those awkward spots at the back of the shoulders, up and down the spine and across the lower back. Use with soap or body shampoo.

HAND PROBLEMS

The hand is the most nubile portion of the body, made up of eight bones in the wrist, five in the palm and 14 hinged bones in fingers and thumb. Together they form a delicate mechanism whose movements are controlled by tendons attached to the forearm muscles and to the short and thick muscle in the heel of the palm which operates the thumb. The backs of the hands contain both sebaceous and sweat glands, the palms only sweat glands. They are activated by high temperatures and also by anxiety – we all know of sweaty palms on important occasions; it is easier said than done to "keep cool, calm and collected", but if you do suffer from sweaty hands, avoid strong coffee, tea and other stimulants before an interview.

CHILBLAINS, though more common on the feet, can occur in cold and damp conditions; they are invariably caused by inadequate protection and poor circulation, and by lack of calcium in the diet. Wear warm gloves during winter and speed up the flow of blood by massaging each finger in turn, from the tip down, over the palm and up over the back, using a lubricating cream like Cocoa-Butter Hand and Body Lotion.

Finger exercises improve circulation and help to keep the hands flexible. Clench the fingers tightly to a ball and hold, then open the hands, spreading the fingers wide. Another good exercise consists in keeping the hands limp and relaxed from the wrists, then rotating them slowly, first in one direction, then the other.

SPOTS and brown or "age" stains are usually caused by over-exposure to sun. Unless you wear gloves in summer, protect the hands with PABA Sunscreen. Sensitive skin types are better treated with Body Shop Sensitive Skin Lotion, with soothing extract of lettuce.

CRACKED SKIN Rough, dry skin eventually develops cracks, sometimes deep enough to penetrate the dermis and open the way for germs and inflammation. It can be due to cold weather or rough work, or simply to prolonged neglect. In the first instance, clean out embedded grime with Japanese Washing Grains, bran or oatmeal flakes, followed by a good rub with lemon to remove the stains. Dab the cracks with soothing Sweet Almond Oil, massaging it in gently. Wash the hands well with mild Goat's Milk Soap with Honey and rinse thoroughly in lukewarm water. Dry, then massage the hands with Body Shop Hawthorn Hand Cream, and with Rich Night Cream with Vitamin E before going to bed and pulling on cotton gloves.

HAND PROTECTION

The best cure for hand problems is prevention of the circumstances that cause them: water, detergents, household chemicals and environmental factors. That is, of course, impossible, but we can still protect our hands to some extent and make up for the rest with daily care. Whenever possible, wear gloves: cotton ones in summer, woollen ones in winter; for all household work use cotton-lined rubber gloves, and for gardening and other rough work a pair of reinforced fabric gloves.

Failing gloves, use a good barrier cream over hands and wrists and reapply it every time the hands have been in water. Use a mild soap for cleansing and be sure to rinse it off properly and to dry thoroughly, especially between the fingers; rashes are caused not so much by rings as by soap and/or detergents trapped in them. **Treat the hands to cream after every wash.**

Once a week at least, give the hands a good soak in warmed Almond Oil, followed by a massage with Hawthorn Hand Cream, and cotton gloves for the night.

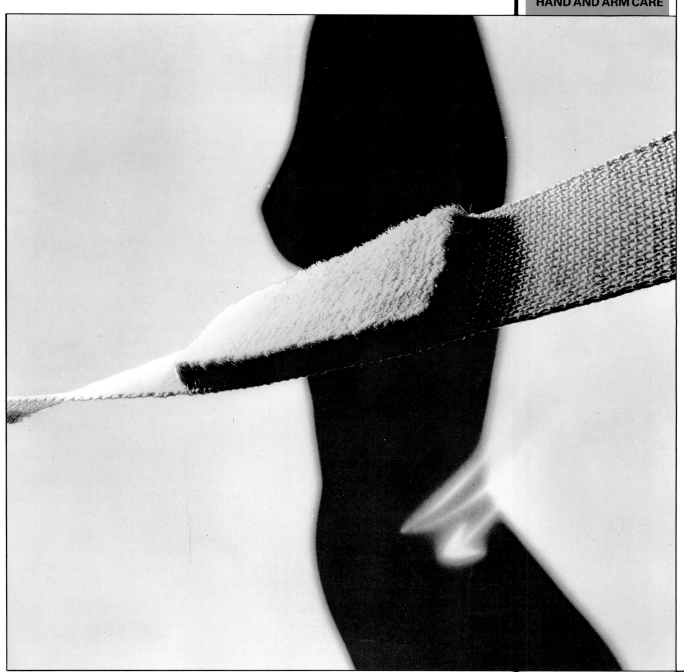

NAIL CARE

Like hair, the visible part of the nail consists of keratin and dead, horny cells. Each nail grows from a bed, known as the matrix, which is overlapped by a thin skin fold or cuticle at the base where the tip of the embryo nail shows as the white half-moon – the rest of the nail extends down to the first finger joint. A shock or blow to the half-moon can cause the nail to grow out discoloured or with a vertical ridge, and if the cuticle is pushed back so as to show a large amount of the half-moon, the soft, jelly-like nail can be damaged by premature exposure to the air.

The growth rate, strength and condition of the nails vary from person to person and are partly determined by inherited genes and partly by nutrition and general state of health. On average, a nail takes five to six months to renew itself, though growth is fastest in summer, during pregnancy and through exercises such as typing and piano playing. Growth rate diminishes in winter, during periods of stress and illness, and with age; there is some evidence that the contraceptive pill also inhibits nail growth.

NAIL PROBLEMS

Healthy nails depend, like other body components, on a diet adequate in protein, vitamins and essential minerals, and trace elements, notably zinc and iodine. A lack of any of these show up on the nails; BRITTLE AND SPLITTING nails indicate lack of vitamin A (or retinol). External factors can also cause brittle nails; detergents, disinfectants, the chlorine in swimming-pool water, harsh soaps and lotions, and incorrect manicure can all be responsible.

HANGNAILS, when a piece of the epidermis is torn away from the side or base of the nail so exposing the lower dermis and causing pain, are more likely when the skin is excessively dry. They may also indicate a dietary lack of folic acid. Nails which are pale in colour, instead of the natural pink, and flat and thin probably show lack of iron. The best source of this mineral is liver.

WHITE BANDS AND SPOTS, not due to accidental damage, can be a further complication of weak nails. The likely cause is a deficiency of the trace element zinc which occurs in association with protein, and a lack of vitamin B_6 (pyridoxine). Women who are pregnant or use the contraceptive pill are advised to increase the intake of this vitamin. STAINS on the nails may be due to nicotine, chemical hair dyes, nail hardeners, topical medication and even prolonged stress. The stains will generally disappear as the nails grow out though this may take up to six months. However, the stains can also be caused by strong nail polish removers which strip the surface layer from the nails.

DO-IT-YOURSELF MANICURE

In order to keep nails and cuticles shapely and trim, give them a weekly treatment. As a first step, remove any nail varnish. We do not recommend varnish because it has a drying effect on the nails, but if you must use it, protect the nail surface with a base coat beneath the varnish.

Nail varnish remover is harmful; it dries out the nails, and pure acetone in particular can strip off the surface layer and cause the nails to flake. Use an oil-based remover, as rarely as possible, wiping off the varnish from the base of the nail towards the tip to prevent it from damaging the cuticle. In between manicures, repair any chips with varnish, and do not chip or peel off varnish with a sharp instrument.

If you have the time, soften nails and cuticles for half an hour in a bowl of warm water and body shampoo. Next file the nails into shape, rounded ovals rather than points which are liable to breaking. Avoid metal files which can cause splitting and flaking; stick to emery boards, using the smooth side to file from the edges towards the centre, and holding it at an angle of 45° to the nail. Do not file too low at the corners of the nails as this weakens growth, and do not use scissors. A damaged nail can be cut straight across with nail clippers and smoothed with the emery board.

After filing, clean under the nails with an orange stick tipped with cottonwool and finish off the filing by bevelling the edges lightly with the smooth side of the emery board. Massage a cuticle cream or oil into the cuticle and round the sides of the nails; avoid chemical cuticle removers – and nail strengtheners – containing formaldehyde which can damage the nail surface; or rinse it off thoroughly as soon as possible. Gently push the cuticle back with an orange stick covered with cottonwool and work away dead skin at the sides of he nail. **Never use cuticle clippers;** at worst they damage the tender skin fold, making it ripe for infection, and at best they encourage the cuticle to grow more thickly and build up a tissue layer.

Finally, massage the hands, including nails and cuticles, with Body Shop Hawthorn Hand Cream or Cocoa Butter Hand and Body Lotion which contains extract of myrrh for healthy nail growth. If you are going to varnish the nails, you must undo part of the good work and wash the hands to remove all traces of cream from the nails. Apply a coat of acetone-free base coat and let it dry before brushing on the varnish; two or more thin coats· are preferable to one thick layer, and each coat should be allowed to dry before the next is applied. Top with a cover of clear varnish.

LEG AND FOOT CARE

T HE UNDERPINNINGS WHICH SUPPORT AND CARRY THE REST OF our bodies are largely ignored, and yet our general health and looks are dependent on those foundations being in perfect working order. Tired, aching feet and swollen ankles are responsible for many an ageing facial wrinkle and, more importantly, for poor circulation, wrong posture, back and head-aches. The length – and basic shape – of legs and feet is determined by hereditary genes, and there is nothing you can do about those. Exercises, though, to firm and strengthen the leg muscles, and diet and massage to combat fat and cellulite can variously make skinny legs shapelier and slim down flabby ones.

Legs account for about one third of the entire body weight; each leg consists of the thighbone (femur), the longest and strongest of the bones, set into the hip socket at the upper end and into the knee joint at the other; the lower leg, from knee to ankle, contains the thin fibula and the tibia (shinbone); the latter, together with the femur convey the full body weight, through the ankle joint, to the feet where arched bones distribute weight to the heels and toes.

Fact: nail barometers
Your nails are accurate indicators of health; conditions such as rheumatism, poor circulation, heart diseases and hypothyroidism leave their traces on the nails. In underdeveloped countries, doctors diagnose inadequate diets by examining the nails of their patients.

Tip: cuticle softener
Blend together 2 tablespoons pineapple juice, 2 tablespoons egg yolk and ½ teaspoon cider vinegar and soak the nails in it for 30 minutes. Push the cuticles back with an orange stick.

Danger: nail varnish
The colour pigment in varnishes causes yellowing of the nails; always protect the surface with a clear base coat beneath varnish.

119

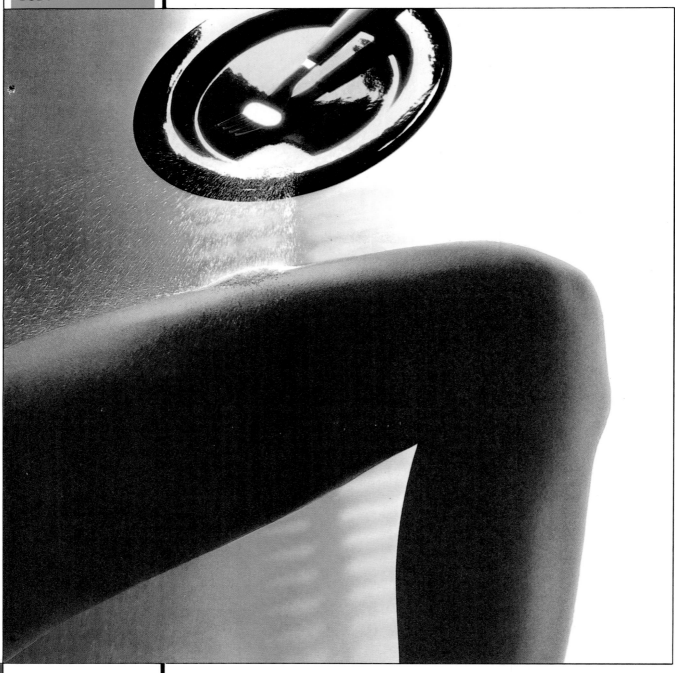

THIGH FLAB

Cellulite is another term for the ugly, rippled bulges on the inside and back of the thighs. Overweight is frequently the cause, but so is restricted circulation from much sitting and tight jeans and girdles, water retention and lack of exercise. Swimming, riding, dancing and bicycling are ideal for keeping the leg muscles in trim, and so are yoga exercises: sitting on the floor, spread the straight legs as far ápart in a fan shape a you can, then slowly bend forward from the waist and clasp the right ankle with the right hand, the left ankle with the left hand. Or simulate bicycling by lying on your back, draw up the knees and, with hips supported by the hands, cycle with the legs in the air. For good leg shape, settle yourself on all fours, back straight, knees and arms rigid; bend one knee forward and bring it up to the chest, then extend it backwards in a straight line. Repeat with the other leg.

Friction massage, during and after a warm bath, is also good, for accelerating cell metabolism and for improving circulation: knead and pinch the fleshy areas and rub vigorously with a loofah, friction glove or Body Buddy. Coarse sea salt on the massage instrument helps to improve skin colour, and Body Shop's Anti-Cellulite Oil is specially formulated to break down the fatty tissues.

Always massage upwards in the direction of the heart. Alternate sprays of hot and cold water can also be effective in dispersing cellulite on thighs and buttocks.

THE LOWER LEG

Apart from flabby muscles, flaky, dry skin and superfluous hair are the most common problems. Lotions and creams on the dry areas are of little use unless the dead skin is first sloughed off. Dead skin accumulates especially on the legs because they are clothed in tight nylon stockings and jeans and seldom exposed to fresh air. Make a habit of exfoliating the legs at bathtime several times a week, rubbing briskly upwards with a loofah or friction glove. Japanese Washing Grains, oatmeal or coarse salt will deal with the more stubborn areas; rinse off thoroughly, then massage with body or aromatherapy oils or with rich lanolin cream.

Unwanted hair on the legs can be removed by temporary shaving and chemical depilation or by permanent electrolysis, but waxing is the most satisfactory treatment, as the hairs are pulled out by the roots and regrowth is slow and fine. The Body Shop Leg Wax has a soothing honey base.

VARICOSE VEINS

These are not only disfiguring, they also pose potential health hazards. The blood vessels in the legs are under continuous strain because the blood flow back to the heart operates against gravity; if the valves in the veins fail to work properly, the veins begin to bulge where the incoming and backflowing blood meet. They become blue in colour and twist into permanent knots which in severe cases can cause ulcers and thrombosis. Varicose veins cannot cure themselves but need medical and/or surgical intervention, involving the removal of a badly affected vein, with no guarantee that another vein will not suffer a similar affliction. Some people are predisposed to varicose veins, but primarily the condition is caused by lack of activity of the leg muscles. Overweight, much standing and pregnancy are all contributary factors; walk as much as possible, massage the legs frequently, always towards the heart, and eat a sensible diet.

Tip: winter legs
Treat rough, flaky skin to a rich massage oil: in a double saucepan melt together 2 tablespoons olive oil and 2 tablespoons lanolin. Blend thoroughly, leave the mixture to cool, then massage it over feet, legs and knees, smoothing it firmly upwards.

Warning: jeans
The rough seams on tight jeans can chafe the skin on the inner thighs and easily lead to broken veins.

Opposite: *A salt rub is marvellous for clearing flaking skin and surface spots. You can use coarse sea salt dry, or you can moisten the skin with warm body oil before rubbing it with a friction glove dipped in salt.*

ANKLES

Some ankles are naturally thick, with firm flesh, and no amount of dieting will slim them down. Obesity is a different matter, and a reducing diet combined with exercises should whittle away the surplus fat in time. Even if you are not overweight ankle exercises help to keep this sensitive joint supple: whenever you are sitting, stretch out the legs and describe 10-12 circles in the air with each foot in turn, from left to right, then in the opposite direction.

Swollen ankles, of a temporary nature, are frequently due to heat or to exhaustion from standing for a long time. You can get immediate relief by putting them up, above hip level in a sitting position and above head level if you lie down. Swelling of the ankles during pregnancy and prior to menstruation is usually due to fluid retention as the body's hormone levels change. Reduce fluid and salt intake in the days just before a period and avoid too many stimulants, such as coffee, tea and alcohol. During pregnancy, put your feet up several times a day, with a pillow beneath them.

Soothe swollen ankles — and tired feet — with a proprietary coolpack or try a simple home treatment of 2 tablespoons of Epsom salts dissolved in 1 litre of lukewarm water; bathe feet and ankles until the ache has eased, then immerse them in cold water to reduce the swelling, pat them dry and then massage gently.

FEET

Think of the constant demands we make on those lowly body components, then consider the minimum care and maintenance we expend on their delicate mechanism — Leonardo da Vinci, who as well as being an artist was also a first-class engineer, called them the finest piece of engineering. Statisticians, who can make figures tell all kinds of tall stories, estimate that the average person walks the equivalent of twice round the world in a lifetime.

The 26 bones in the foot, covered by fine-tuned muscles and tendons and balanced on two main arches (one running from the heel to the base of the little toe, the other from the heel to the big toe), were never designed to be squeezed into tight-fitting shoes, with the heel's balance point suspended in the air.

FOOTWEAR

Shoes are the root of most foot problems, and nylon stockings come a close second. Ideally we should walk barefoot, to let the feet breathe and exercise naturally; whenever you can, peel off shoes and stockings.

Choosing the right shoes is of the utmost importance, and the most expensive are not necessarily the best. No two feet are alike, not even on the same person, but mass-market manufacture is geared to comparatively few shoe lasts. **Never buy shoes in the morning** when the feet are still rested; the afternoon is a much better time. Do try on and walk in BOTH shoes and don't ever assume that you can "break in" a pair of shoes which pinch slightly. High heels may be fashionable, but they are purgatory for your feet, throwing the balance of the whole body forward.

The ideal shoe has a heel no more than 9cm high, supports the instep and fits comfortably round the heel; it should be 1cm longer than the foot and as wide as the broadest point which is at the first joint of the big toe. Avoid plastic which does not allow the feet to breathe, and settle for leather or fabric; don't wear tight boots all day long (they restrict circulation) nor wooden clogs which act like splints.

FOOT EXERCISES

Walk barefoot as often as possible, in order to firm the muscles and to let the feet recover from the confinement of shoes. Practise a few basic exercises:

1. Stand, feet slightly apart, and raise yourself slowly up, then down, with the weight on the toes. Stand and walk on tip toe as often as possible.

2. Stand on the step of a staircase or a thick book, toes extending over the edge; bend the toes as if gripping the edge, hold while counting to two, then pull the toes upwards and hold again to a count of two. Repeat several times, then reverse the position, this time dropping and raising the heels.

3. Sit or lie with feet outstretched; arch one foot at a time and slowly sketch wide circles, first in one direction, then in the other. Repeat several times.

4. Go up the wall, by lying flat on the floor, soles of the feet against the wall, spreading the toes wide as they grasp at the surface. Good against cramp.

FOOT PROBLEMS

Many of these are caused by bad-fitting shoes or inadequate foot care. Blisters are due to heat friction on pressure points such as the heels, the instep and on the outer side of the soles. Protect them with adhesive padding, before they burst and until they have healed. CORNS are by far the most common, frequently on the toe joints and are again formed by friction and pressure. The skin reacts by building up a hard, pointed layer of dead skin cells. **Never** attempt to cut or otherwise treat a corn; it

Warning: chilblains
Common on feet in cold, damp conditions and associated with poor circulation. Massage in foot lotion while the feet are still cold to avoid chilblains. Exercise regularly and wear comfortable shoes.

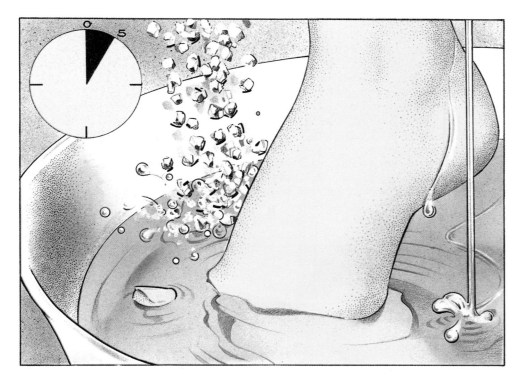

A foot bath revives tired and swollen feet. Soothe them for 5-10 minutes in warm water softened with Epsom salt, bath crystals, gel or aromatherapy oil, then revive them with a quick dip into cold water before drying, creaming and massaging them.

needs professional attention by a chiropodist. CALLOUSES are similar to corns but flat rather than rounded and therefore less painful.

BUNIONS are painful deformities of the big toe, caused by weak or slack muscles at the joint with the metatarsal bone. They may be inherited or be due to bad footwear. In severe cases, surgery is the only remedy.

WARTS and VERRUCAE may look like corns or callouses, but differ in being alive and moist and in having a blood supply. They are caused by a virus, warts often spreading to clusters and verrucae growing inwards. It is essential to treat the virus, as well as the symptoms, preferably by a foot specialist.

ATHLETE'S FOOT is a fungal infection encouraged by hot weather and moist skin; it is easily picked up and spread in communal gyms and swimming pools. Symptoms include itching and rashes, splitting and peeling of the skin between the toes and blisters under them. You can prevent athlete's foot by carefully washing the feet after a visit to public swimming baths, drying them well and wearing cotton socks and open sandals which do not easily collect moisture.

INGROWING TOE NAILS can be excruciating. They are caused by incorrect nail cutting and/or too narrow shoes, and unless they are treated early they tend to recur, growing ever deeper and more painfully into the skin.

DO-IT-YOURSELF PEDICURE

The daily bathing routine obviously extends to the feet; wash them in soap and warm water and dry thoroughly. A little extra attention will pay off: exfoliate them at least once a week with a bristle brush or pumice stone over hard-skin areas; massage them briskly with Peppermint Foot Lotion, which soothes the feet, softens hard skin, dispels foot odour and protects against chilblains.

Once every 10 or 14 days give your feet a pedicure, following basically the same procedure as for a manicure:

1. Having removed old varnish, soak the feet in warm water for 5-10 minutes. You can add Epsom salts to relax them and a few frops of camphor oil for sweaty feet.

2. Trim the nails with clippers, cutting them straight across and slightly longer than the tips of the toes, to prevent ingrowing nails. Smooth the edges with an emery board and massage toes and nails with Peppermint Foot Lotion.

3. Clean under the nails with an orange stick tipped with cottonwool. Push the cuticles gently back and buff the nails to gloss and stimulate them.

4. Massage feet and ankles, with sweeping movement, using Body Shop Cocoa-Butter Hand and Body Lotion, Rich Massage or Peppermint Foot Lotion.

5. Finally, apply a base coat, followed by two thin coats of varnish and top with a clear, protective layer. If you sweep a curve from the base of the cuticle, outwards towards the sides and inwards towards the nail tip, with a straight central stroke, the nail will appear to be oval in shape.

AROMATHERAPY & MASSAGE

AROMATHERAPY

CELLULITE

MASSAGE

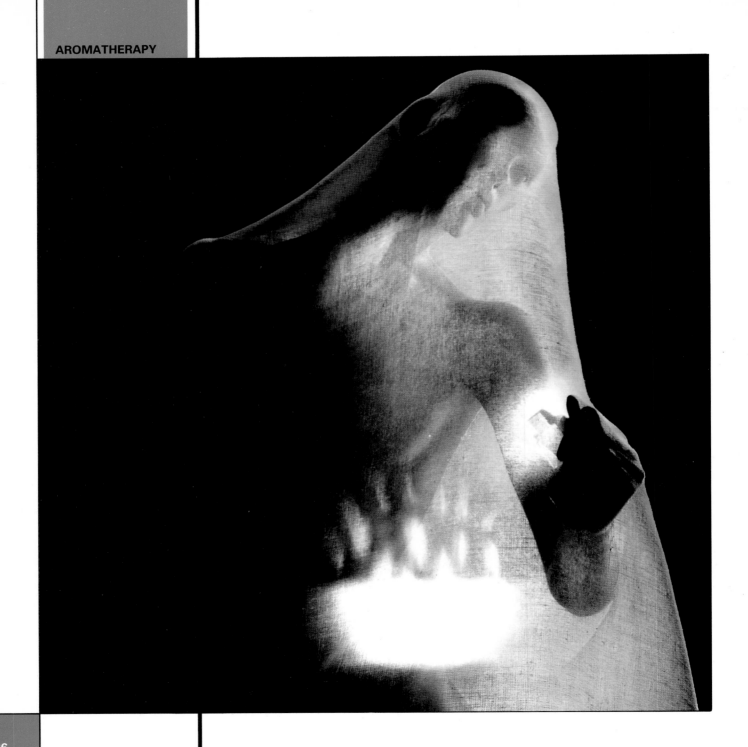

AROMATHERAPY

AROMATHERAPY IS THE PRACTICE OF USING OILS EXTRACTED FROM aromatic plants to enhance health and appearance. Essential oils contain the scent of the flowers, leaves, stems, roots or bark from which they come and have been used as perfumes for thousands of years. Apart from their pleasing aromas, essential oils are valued equally for their potent cosmetic and therapeutic properties. They are said to soothe away tension, improve concentration and lift depression, and to fight infection, speed healing and reduce inflammation. Aromatherapy is perhaps the most luxurious treatment for mind and body.

THE HISTORY OF AROMATHERAPY

The ancient Chinese are generally acknowledged as the founders of aromatherapy, but it is more than likely that quite early in the history of civilization man had realized that certain aromatic plants could help restore his health. We know that traditional Indian medicine (*Ayur Veda*), which goes back 3000 years, describes healing and rejuvenation formulas that incorporate essential oils.

The use of aromatic substances certainly flourished with the Egyptians. During the times of the pharaohs splendid botanical gardens were created along the banks of the Nile and stocked with medicinal plants, many of which were collected from places like Arabia, the Indes and Malaysia. In 1500 BC Pharaoh Thotmes III (Tuthmosis III) sent an expedition to Syria in search of new healing plants. Paintings of these plants can be seen on the walls of the temple at Karnak, dedicated to the deity Aman, and later on the tomb of Tutankhamun. Translations of hieroglyphics on papyri and steles found in ancient tombs and temples reveal that aromatics were used to treat a variety of illnesses. The temple priests were the physicians of the day, who formulated and prepared medicinal concoctions of essential oils. They also used the oils for embalming, for creating perfumes for the pharaohs and for scenting the temples during religious ceremonies.

Greek physicians visited Egypt and brought back an increased knowledge of essential oils. Recipes for medicinal perfumes are inscribed on marble tablets in the temples of Aesculapius, the Greek god of healing, and of Aphrodite, the goddess of love. Marestheus, a renowned physician, noted that aromatic plants, especially flowers, often possessed stimulating or edifying properties. He cited rose, and other fruity and spicy scents, as being invigorating for a tired mind. The Romans also used perfumed oils chiefly to scent themselves and their surroundings.

In the 10th century the Arabs were extracting essential oils from aromatic plants and using them medicinally. The Knights of the Crusades brought aromatic essences and waters back to Europe from the Middle East and they became so popular that perfume began to be manufactured and was well established by the end of the 12th century. The importance of aromatic plants for other purposes was realized early. When the bubonic plague reached England around the middle of the 14th century,

---

Hint: anxiety?
The emotional and the physical are so closely linked that anxiety or fear may cause an attack of asthma or stomach ache. Treat the emotion, and the physical discomfort will often disappear.

Fact or fiction?
In Greek mythology, Venus is said to be the first user of aromatics. Her secrets were revealed to mankind by her handmaiden Aenore. Paris handed them on to Helen of Troy, whose fabled beauty caused the siege and fall of Troy.

Opposite: *Aromatherapy is more than massage, for the essential oils which bring relief to aching muscles also calm the senses, instilling tranquility to body and mind. Added to a steam bath or wafted across a room, the effect is instant and lasting.*

Warning: lemon oil
Lemons manufacture citral, one of the main components of essential oils. The trees flourish in Sicily, where a manufacturing plant now operates. The reason: it takes more than 3000 lemons to yield 1 kg of essential oil; the synthetic version is both cheaper and easier to produce.

fires were ordered in the streets at night, burning aromatic frankincense and pine; indoors, incense and perfumed candles were burnt to combat infection and disguise the stench of death; pomanders made from aromatic gums and resins were worn on ribbons round the neck to protect the wearers from the dreaded Black Death.

By the turn of the 18th century essential oils were widely used in medicinal preparations and Salmon's Dispensary of 1896 contains recipes for numerous aromatic remedies. In the 19th century, essential oils were subjected to more scientific investigation, and it was discovered that some of them could be synthesized from other materials. As it is always quicker and cheaper to produce the laboratory versions than natural plant extractions, true essential oils began to fall from favour. Today, many of our medicines and perfumes contain so-called essential oils, though often they are mere imitations; while synthetics may smell like the real thing, they do not possess the same therapeutic properties.

Dr Jean Valnet, a French doctor who used essential oils during the Second World War in the treatment of wounds and infections, firmly believed that natural essential oils are infinitely superior in their action to any synthetic product. His beliefs were shared by Madame Marguerite Maury, a biochemist who worked with Valnet. She suggested that essential oils could be beneficial in skin care and she was particularly intrigued by the prospect that they might help to delay the ageing process and solve problems caused by stress. It is upon her work that most modern aromatherapy treatments are based.

ESSENTIAL OILS
Essential oils are highly scented droplets found in minute quantities in the flowers, stems, leaves, roots and barks of aromatic plants. They are not true oils in the manner of lubricant vegetable oils, but highly fluid and exceptionally volatile: be careful not to leave the top off the containers as essential oils do evaporate.

Essential oils are complex mixtures of different organic molecules – terpenes, alcohols, esters, aldehydes, ketones and phenols. Synthetic oils are usually made from one or more of the constituents predominant within a particular essential oil; menthol, for example, often substitutes for mint and eucalyptol for eucalyptus. However, there are sound reasons for believing that it is the interaction between each and every component that gives an essential oil its particular character and unique therapeutic properties.

The chemical composition of an oil is related to the time of day, the month or the season. Jasmine develops a strongly scented indole molecule at midnight when it is particularly intoxicating, and it is important to gather the petals at exactly the right moment. There are good years and bad years for essential oils as there are with wines. Some commercial producers have discovered that they can improve the quality of a poor yield by adding certain components and that an expensive oil like rosemary can be adulterated, without altering its aroma, by adding 30-40% of camphor which is considerably cheaper for the perfume industry. Such adulteration may be commercially acceptable but it might well alter the therapeutic properties of the oil. We try to ensure that our essential oils come from reputable sources and are as pure as possible.

Experts recognize an essential oil by its aroma and check its composition by a process called Gas Liquid Chromatography. Colour can also be an indicator;

eucalyptus is colourless, chamomile varies from white to blue and others, like basil and sandalwood (both light greenish-yellow), are in pastel shades. Yet others are richly pigmented, like jasmine, a deep reddish-brown, patchouli, brown, and rose, orange-red.

EXTRACTION OF THE OILS

Essential oils may be extracted from plants in a number of ways. One of the oldest methods is distillation, practised in ancient Persia, Turkey and India thousands of years ago. The Egyptians were preparing essence of cedarwoods for embalming and other purposes around 2000 BC; the wood was heated in a clay vessel covered by a screen of woollen fibres through which the steam had to pass. The essence was obtained by squeezing out the impregnated wool.

The Arab physician, Avicenna, is credited with having popularized distillation in the late 10th century. He began with extract of rose petals then experimented with other aromatic materials. Today, distillation remains the most commonly used means of extracting essential oils.

Other methods include *enfleurage*, often used for delicate petals like jasmine and tuberose; maceration, for tougher flowers and leaves, roots and bark; solvent extraction, the preferred method for gums and resins like myrrh and galbanum; and hand expression, chiefly employed for squeezing the highly aromatic oils from thick-skinned citrus fruit like oranges, tangerines and lemons.

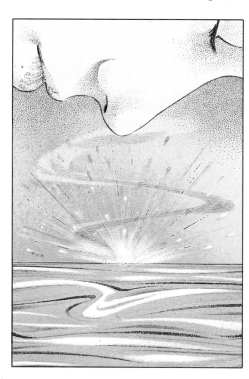

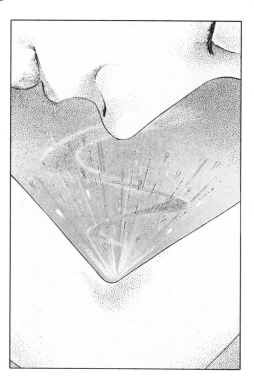

Warning: fakes
If you are not sure that the essential oil you are thinking of buying is pure, let price be the guide. Pure, undiluted essential oils can cost several pounds sterling – and upwards – for a 15ml bottle.

Tip: storing oils
Essential oils owe their elusiveness to a high number of free electrons. To preserve their properties, essential oils must be stored in airtight, dark glass bottles, away from direct sunlight.

Essential oils *are contained as minute droplets in flowers (far left), their scent most heady at night, and in the barks of such tropical evergreens as the camphor and cinnamon trees.*

BODY SHOP ESSENTIAL OILS				
TYPE OF OIL	USES	METHOD OF APPLICATION	FREQUENCY	COMMENTS
CHAMOMILE	Dry sensitive skins Ideal for children	Baths, massage Facial massage	As often as needed Daily	Good for allergic skins Calms children
EUCALYPTUS	Improves breathing Helps relieve muscular and rheumatic pains	Chest and throat massage, inhalation Baths, massage over specific areas	As often as needed	Fresh and invigorating, mildly analgesic
LAVENDER	Sensitive skins Relaxation	Facial massage Inhalation, baths, massage	Daily Nightly, whenever tense	Excellent for problem skins Ideal for physical and mental tension
NEROLI	Dry, irritated skins Relaxation	Facial massage Baths, massage	Daily Nightly	Calming to skins Anti-depressant
PEPPERMINT	Hot, sticky skin Improves breathing	Bath and body massage Inhalation	After sunbathing Twice daily	Cooling effect on skin Clears breathing and nasal passages
ROSE	Mature, dry and puffy skins Relaxation	Facial massage Body massage	Daily Daily	Soothing and antiseptic Marvellous perfume oil
TANGERINE	All skins during pregnacy Good for children Helps improve energy levels	Massage Baths, massage	Whenever needed, daily during pregnancy As needed	Energizing; great as a pick-me-up after illnesses

THE PROPERTIES AND USES OF ESSENTIAL OILS

Essential oils possess numerous properties which make them useful for treating many of our most common health and beauty troubles. We rarely realize how strongly the smells that surround us affect the way we feel. We perfume our bodies and scent our rooms with fresh flowers or potpourri because they give us – and hopefully others – pleasure. We never stop to wonder why.

Professor Paolo Rovesti, Director of the Instituto Derivati Vegetali in Milan, has studied the effect of essential oils on the psyche and found that they can be useful in the treatment of anxiety and depression. He recommends ylang-ylang, citrus oils, jasmine, basil, patchouli and peppermint for treating general depression, geranium, lavender and bergamot for treating fear and anxiety, and peppermint, rose and carnation for improving concentration and eliminating lethargy. Sprayed into the air, these oils also have immediate and long-lasting effects.

The reasons for these reactions are as yet unclear, but it is known that odour molecules are perceived by thousands of tiny nerve cells in the nose and that each of these nerves is connected to that part of the brain which is concerned with emotional drives, creativity and sexual behaviour. This could explain why certain perfumes make us feel happy, why some essences, like jasmine and rose, have a reputation for being aphrodisiac and why unpleasant smells, like petrol fumes, can induce depression. While pure essential oils appear to have a positive influence on the psyche, it is doubtful that synthetic ones work in the same way.

Myth or fact?
Soothe depressing moods with essential oils:
Melancholy – rose, neroli or chamomile.
Anxiety – chamomile, neroli, or lavender.
Anger – rose or chamomile
Impatience – chamomile or lavender.
Suspicion – lavender.

Refreshing tip:
Tangerine oil's revitalizing qualities help restore health after illness. Also good for massaging children and a soothing back massage for anxiety or for pregnant mothers.

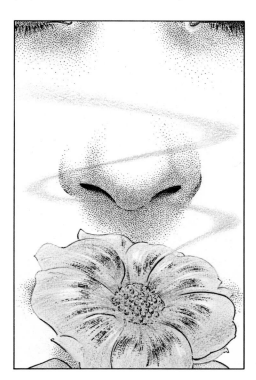

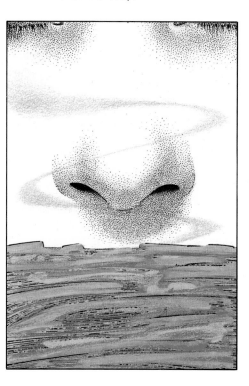

Sensory or sensuous, *essential oils like eucalyptus and peppermint ease laboured breathing (far left); a few drops of rose oil in the crook of an arm arouse the senses.*

The aroma of pure essential oils appears to trigger off psychological responses to overcome emotional tension (below). Almost visibly, facial aromatherapy smoothes out the crumpled look of depression (left), relaxes the stretch marks of anxiety and restores tone to muscles distorted in concentration (right).

SOOTHING THE NERVES

Essential oils are valued for the effect they have on the nervous system. The autonomic nervous system is divided into two parts, the sympathetic and the parasympathetic nerves, both operating below the level of consciousness. They work in opposition. The sympathetic branch is concerned with the active, dynamic state, which is necessary for movement and accomplishment. The parasympathetic branch conserves energy, relaxes the body, helping it to recuperate during sleep and holidays. The two branches are designed to work in harmony to maintain a perfect balance in the body; however, depending on the life-style we lead, the balance can be upset, and we end up feeling tense or lethargic.

Essential oils work to redress the imbalance between the two branches and they often have dual functions. Someone suffering from fatigue as a result of nervous tension can be calmed and stimulated at the same time by smelling peppermint. Few drugs can claim to work in this way. Tranquilisers may calm the system so that you end up feeling fatigued and fit for nothing but bed.

Essential oils are useful for treating stress-linked problems, ranging from digestive upsets, allergies and tension headaches, to insomnia and skin eruptions.

Neroli oil, one of the more expensive oils, is a potent sedative and anti-depressant, acting via the nervous system to give calmness and tranquility. Some describe its effect as almost hypnotic. It also acts beneficially on the skin and is reputed to be good for treating dryness and for using over broken veins.

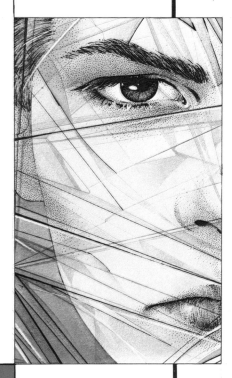
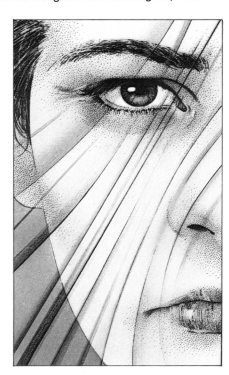
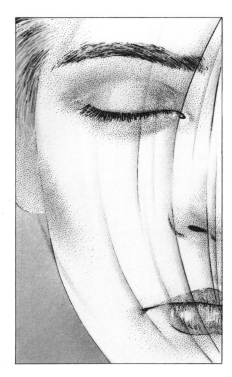

FIGHTING INFECTION

The ancient Egyptians must have been aware that essential oils possessed anti-bacterial properties because they used them for embalming the dead. The essences could preserve the flesh of the mummies by halting the putrifying action of bacteria. Early Greek physicians had the same knowledge. When an epidemic plague broke out in Athens (c 430BC), Hippocrates urged the inhabitants to burn aromatic plants in the streets to protect themselves and prevent the plague from spreading.

The first research into the antiseptic powers of essential oils was carried out by Chamberland in 1887. He found that cinnamon, angelica and geranium were active in preventing the growth and proliferation of anthrax bacilli. Later work substantiated his findings and classified essential oils according to their antiseptic powers. One of the most potent antiseptics is eucalyptus which contains the powerfully anti-bacterial constituent, eucalyptol; others are lemon, pine, clove, thyme and cinnamon. Such antiseptic properties make them useful for treating coughs, colds and flu, and for preventing them in winter by surrounding yourself with these essential oils which will help to bolster the body's resistance.

Chamomile is one of the most soothing oils known, particularly for children; it is used for treating external inflammatory conditions and helps to dispel stomach discomfort and soothe aches and pains in joints and muscles.

The same anti-bacterial properties are useful for treating the skin, cleansing infected wounds and helping to keep spots at bay. Spots materialise when oil or sebum gets trapped in the follicle and bacterial activity leads to irritation of the lining of the follicle. This in turn becomes inflamed and infected, resulting in a spot. Essential oils help to prevent spot formation and encourage existing spots to clear up quickly by keeping the bacteria under control.

NATURE'S HEALERS

The story goes that a chemist called Rene Maurice Gattefosse was working in his laboratory when a small explosion seriously burnt his hands. He plunged them into a jar of neat lavender oil which happened to be close by on the desk, and was amazed at how quickly they healed without any apparent scarring. Following this finding he made use of the healing properties of essential oils in his surgery during the 1914-1918 war. Gattefosse actually coined the term aromatherapy to describe the therapeutic use of aromatic oils.

Essential oils appear to work by speeding up the process of cellular regeneration, making the skin heal faster. The process of cell renewal slows down as we get older; it was the Austrian biochemist, Marguerite Maury, who suggested that essential oils applied to the skin might speed up cell renewal and help preserve a youthful appearance: she was twice awarded the *Prix Internationale d'Esthétique et Cosmétologie* for her work.

Certain essential oils also help to reduce inflammation and they are particularly beneficial for treating sore cuts, burns and bruises. Their anti-inflammatory properties also make them useful for relieving the pain of arthritis and rheumatism, both inflammatory conditions affecting joints, bones, muscles and joint linings. Thyme, sage and rosemary are reputed to be especially anti-inflammatory. Injuries, such as sprained ankles, torn ligaments and "tennis elbow", can all be treated with essential oils, as can aches and pains from stiff muscles.

Tip: winter colds
Scent your surroundings as protection against bacteria: add a few drops of peppermint oil to a bowl of warm water and place it on a table away from the window. Or drop them on to a piece of damp cottonwool placed on a radiator.

Beauty hint:
To clear blemished skin, place two drops each of chamomile and lavender oil (ready diluted) into the palm of your hand. Rub the hands together to mix the essences and massage them into the skin in the evening after cleansing the skin thoroughly; leave on overnight.

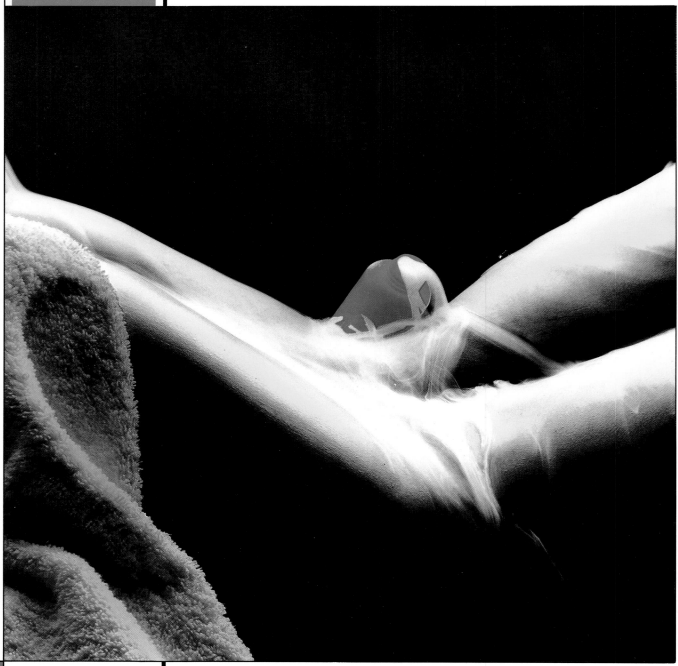

REVITALIZERS

It would appear that essential oils affect the body's hormone-producing glands. Research has shown that after entering the bloodstream essential oils can be detected in the glands; some essential oils remain longer in an ailing organ than in a healthy one, and certain oils seem to be attracted to specific organs. Violet leaf oil, for example, was found in greater concentration in the kidney than elsewhere in the body, while rose oil was found mainly in the ovaries.

It is thought that essential oils do not home in on the organs, but that the organs themselves absorb the oils as they do other nutrients. Dr Valnet suggests that pine, sage, rosemary and geranium have the ability to galvanize the adrenal cortex (layer) and alleviate tension caused by stress. Anise and mint stimulate the pituitary gland, which in turn affects most of the other hormone-producing glands. Some oils help to regulate the menstrual cycle and can be used to treat pre-menstrual tension, irregular menstruation, amenorrhoea (absence of menstruation) and menopausal problems. Others, such as cinnamon and ylang-ylang, are said to revive a waning interest in sex.

MASSAGE

Essential oils are probably best used in massage. Neat oils must be diluted in a carrier oil before being applied to the skin or they will cause irritation. The carrier can be any kind of vegetable oil – almond, grape seed and sunflower are some of the best. Body Shop Aromatherapy Oils are already diluted and ready for use, being 3% concentrations of essential oils in almond oil.

Smooth, firm massage strokes (effleurage) are best as they warm the skin and aid the penetration of essential oils; vigorous hacking and squeezing should be avoided, the aim of the massage should be to promote relaxation and ease the entry of the oils. These probably enter the body through the pores that secrete sweat and sebum, then diffuse into the blood capillaries and intercellular fluid and travel round the body in the lymph and blood.

Total absorption takes from 10 to 100 minutes, depending on the essential oils. Never shower straight after the skin has been massaged with an aromatherapy oil.

BATH OILS AND VAPORIZERS

Essential oils added to your bath water will penetrate the skin, and as they are highly volatile they will also be carried in the steam. Do keep the bathroom door and windows closed so that you can inhale this therapeutic vapour. For best effects, add about ten drops of diluted essential oil to a bath. Rose Oil, from the fragrant damask rose, is an expensive oil, but highly antiseptic and soothing for nervous and pre-menstrual tension and as an overall tonic. Lavender is one of the most versatile of essential oils, relieving all kinds of tension-related problems, balancing the nervous system, steadying the emotions and calming inflammation.

Steaming offers a more direct inhalation than a bath. To make your own vapourizer, half fill a basin with scalding water, lean over the basin with your face about 20cm from the surface. Cover your head with a towel, and add five drops of oil. Both Peppermint and Eucalyptus Oil are ideal for vaporizing; menthol and eucalyptol respectively are excellent for treating respiratory and sinus problems. They also have a cooling effect on tissues and tired muscles. *The Body Shop does not recommend the ingestion of aromatherapy oils.*

Tip: aches and pains
For the relief of muscular pains, massage the afflicted areas with 6 drops of eucalyptus and 6 drops of lavender oil, mixed together in an eggcup.

Tips: bath oils
For an invigorating morning bath, add 2 drops of rose, 2 drops of tangerine and 6 drops of lavender oil to a tub of hot water. For a relaxing evening bath, add 2 drops of camomile, 2 drops of rose and 6 drops of lavender oil.

Opposite: *Revitalizing oils affect the body's hormone balance, leaving on the skin an enveloping aroma as refreshing as gentle foam.*

Warning: posture
Poor posture places undue stress and strain on muscles, interfering with the flow of circulation, particularly to the lower half of the body. Walk tall to minimize the risk of cellulite.

Danger: nicotine
Smoking is the cellulite sufferer's worst enemy. Nicotine impedes the absorption of vitamins and impairs the circulation. Carbon monoxide takes the place of nourishing oxygen in the blood, and nicotine constricts the blood capillaries that feed the tissues.

Opposite: *Rose oil, most exquisite of all, has been valued since the ancient Greeks first extracted the precious drops from fragrant damask roses and suspended them in water.*

CELLULITE

LTHOUGH THE WORD "CELLULITE" DOES NOT APPEAR IN ANY dictionary, medical or otherwise, there must be few women who have not heard about it. Variously referred to as "orange peel skin" or "jodpur thighs", cellulite is the lumpy flesh commonly found on the buttocks and thighs and, to a lesser extent, on the stomach, upper arms and knees. Because cellulite is not recognized by the British Medical Association, your doctor may insist that this ugly condition is nothing more than plain fat. The fact that cellulite is not cured by calorie-controlled diets and that it can be found on the slimmest of women has prompted scientists, mainly in France and Italy, to study the complaint in depth. Their findings indicate that cellulite differs from ordinary fat, in physiological terms and in appearance. Where cellulite is found, the underlying tissue structure appears to be distorted. Close examination reveals that the tiny blood vessels which weave their way between the fat cells seem to be particularly permeable. Consequently, fluid leaks from them and seeps into the spaces between the cells. This "water-logging" makes the skin look puffy and, more importantly, interferes with the flow of blood to the area. As a result, the delivery to the cells of nutrients on the one hand and excretion of waste products on the other are both slowed down. Apparently irritated by the build-up of toxic wastes, collagen fibrils thicken and wrap themselves round the fat cells. Micro-nodules are formed, which can later regroup into macro-nodules, effectively locking the fat away and making it difficult to shift by diet alone.

Macro-nodules can be felt as tiny lumps just under the surface of the skin; they are responsible for giving skin that unsightly "orange peel" look when gently squeezed.

THE HORMONE LINK
The causes that trigger the cellulite conditon are unknown, but statistics reveal that in 75% of cases, its appearance coincides with a major hormonal upheaval in the body. While 12% of cellulite appears at puberty, 17% occurs during pregnancy, 19% in association with the contraceptive pill, and 27% of cases result at the beginning of the menopause.

High levels of the female hormone, oestrogen, can cause water retention by acting on the permeability of the blood capillaries. This could help to explain why cellulite becomes more noticeable just before a period is due. It also sheds light on why men, no matter how obese, rarely get cellulite.

THE STRESS FACTOR
Women often get cellulite or find that cellulite becomes more obvious during prolonged periods of stress or emotional trauma. This is because stress acts directly on the hypothalamus in the brain, which in turns sends signals to its second-in-command, the pituitary gland, often called the "master" gland, which probably

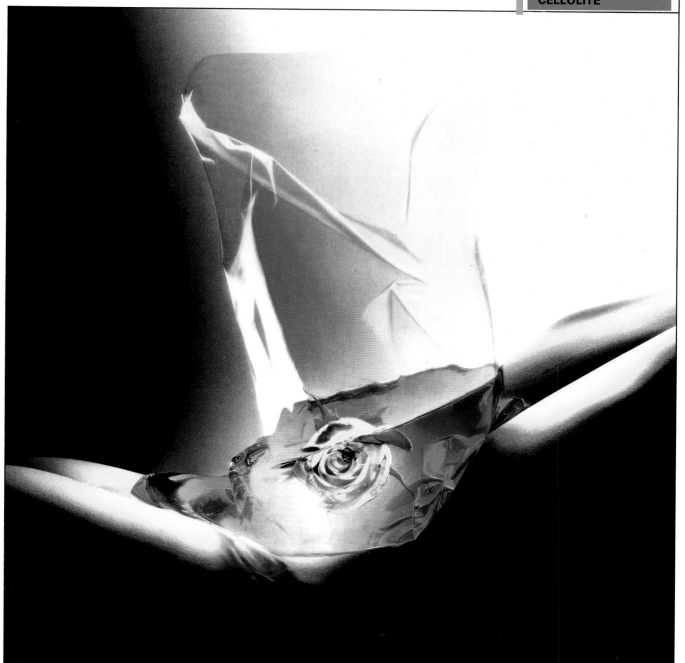

orchestrates the activities of all the other hormone-producing glands. The well-known fact that anxiety can upset the menstrual cycle, causing a period to be early or late, is a clear example of how emotions can disrupt hormone levels.

Stress also triggers off the production of an anti-diuretic hormone which causes fluid to be retained in the tissues. This explains why we often feel bloated when we are anxious or frightened. Although for the most part unconsciously, we contract certain muscles when we are under stress. Tense muscles impede the free flow of blood and lymph round the body, and poor circulation is thought to contribute to the development of cellulite.

THE CIRCULATION AND LYMPATHIC CONNECTIONS

Poor circulation, whether inherited or due to lack of activity, is undoubtedly involved in the formation of cellulite. Stagnation of blood in certain areas is known to create conditions condusive to the development of those immovable pockets of fat and water. The fact that the skin invariably feels cold to the touch, where cellulite lurks, substantiates the notion that circulation in these tissues is sluggish.

Exercise is one of the best ways of improving general circulation, but massage is preferable for stimulating the blood flow in certain tissues.

Massage also helps to prevent and banish cellulite by improving the flow of lymph, the colourless fluid, packed with white blood cells, that picks up metabolic wastes and other toxins from the cells and transports them to other areas for disposal. When lymphatic drainage is sluggish the fluid lingers in certain areas, making the skin look puffy. The build-up of toxins in the tissues also sets up conditions that induce the formation of cellulite; if it is already present they simply aggravate the condition.

Lymph is pumped round the body by contraction of the lymph vessels and by the contraction and relaxation of the surrounding muscles, together with the suction created when we breathe. Gentle, rhythmic stretching exercises, like yoga, are therefore helpful for combatting cellulite.

THE FOOD FACTOR

While dieting on its own will not shift cellulite, a lowered calorie intake is still essential in order to mobilize excess fat from the cells. How efficiently this fat can be removed from the tissues will depend on blood and lymph flow, as well as on the state of the collagen fibrils that wrap themselves round the fat cells. These tissues can be radically affected by massage.

The kind of food we eat may play a role in the formation of cellulite. Salt acts like a magnet to water, causing it to be retained in the tissues. Avoid salted nuts and crisps, processed foods like bacon and salami, and most canned and packaged foods.

Fresh fruits and green leafy vegetables have a high fibre content and should help in the fight against cellulite, because they have a cleansing effect on the body tissues. Berry and citrus fruit are also a good source of the important vitamin C.

The liver is the organ primarily responsible for neutralizing toxins within the body. Overloading the liver with rich, fatty and creamy foods, chemical additives, caffeine (present in coffee, coca-cola and tea) and alcohol can prevent it from doing its job properly. As a result, irritant wastes linger in the tissues where they can encourage cellulite formation.

THE FLUID FACTOR

It might be thought that taking in lots of water could serve only to worsen the problem of fluid retention in the tissues. However, the reverse seems to be true; six to eight glasses of pure, unadulterated spring or mineral water seem to help keep cellulite at bay, probably because water helps the kidneys to flush toxins out of the body. Some proprietary mineral waters also have a diuretic action, encouraging the body to shed excess fluids.

MASSAGE FOR CELLULITE

If you want to banish cellulite, and banish it for good, massage is an important part of your daily routine. It is primarily designed to improve lymphatic drainage, but will also stimulate blood flow through the tissues. Set aside 5 minutes, morning and evening, to stroke the body from head to toe with a dry sisal brush. Use long sweeping movements and firm, but not hard pressure, to brush from the tips of the fingers up the arms. Then brush down the neck, across the shoulders, and down the breasts. Sweep down the back and down the tummy and finally work from the toes, up the front and back of the legs and up over the buttocks. **Do not rub back or forth or use circular movements.**

During a bath or shower work the affected areas with a Body Buddy; the specially moulded nodules encourage the softening of collagen fibrils and increase fat mobilization without the need to apply too much pressure. These problem areas tend to be painful to the touch, and they bruise easily if zealously attacked.

After a bath, when the skin is warm and the muscles relaxed, massage the cellulite with your hands. Begin with the effleurage technique to stimulate circulation, then take hold of the flesh with both hands and squeeze, first with one hand, then the other, working over the whole area. Clench your hands and push the knuckles into the skin, twisting them around at the same time. Finally stroke the area again with the Body Buddy, always working towards the heart.

MAJJAGE

MASSAGE CAN BE DESCRIBED AS THE ART OF TOUCHING. AT ITS most rudimentary, it is a silent, but expressive form of communication between two persons. There is no better way of comforting and showing that you care than laying a reassuring hand on someone's shoulder or touching a cheek. The more complex, structured systems of massage touching go much further: they are invaluable for helping to relieve tension, alleviate fatigue and instil deep relaxation, and they encourage the body's organs and systems to function optimally and speed the healing of damaged tissues. Discover massage and you will have found a means of enhancing the health and vitality of yourself – and perhaps others – and of acquiring better self knowledge.

Tip: salt rub
Before a massage, slough off dead skin to activate circulation. Work coarse sea salt on a flannel over all parts of the body, excepting the face.

TYPES OF MASSAGE

Today's types of massage have their origins in the East. Swedish Massage may not sound particularly Oriental, but nevertheless has its roots in the Far East. It was developed by Per Henrik Ling, a Swede who in the 19th century travelled to China. So impressed was he by the kind of massage practised there, that he synthesized his own system from his knowledge of gymnastics and physiology and the techniques he had observed.

Shiatsu has been practised for centuries in Japan. The complicated system, which centres around energy pathways and pressure points, is based on the principles of traditional Chinese acupuncture; over the years it has been enriched by Western techniques of manipulation, such as osteopathy and chiropractice.

Reflexology, a specialized massage for the hands and feet, is gaining acceptance as a means of diagnosing and treating a variety of minor ills. Paintings discovered on the walls of a physician's tomb in the Valley of the Kings indicate that reflexology, or something very like it, was practised by the ancient Egyptians in 2330 BC. However, it is likely that it stems from the kind of pressure-point therapy that has been used for thousands of years in the Far East.

THE MAGIC OF TOUCH

Most of us underestimate the power of massage, seeing it as a pleasurable experience, but unlikely to change our lives. However, evidence would suggest that massage can profoundly benefit mind and body.

Subconsciously, we rely enormously on our tactile sense for keeping us in touch with reality. Babies and young children first explore the world with their hands; touch is essential for learning and developing. Experiments with monkeys, whose behaviour patterns resemble those of humans, have revealed that without the cuddles and caresses of a caring mother, the young fail to grow healthy and happy. Throughout life we need physical contact in order to feel accepted, secure and loved. When physical contact is withdrawn or lost, we can feel horribly alone and doubt our personal worth.

The British are, sadly, renowned for their reticence about touching one another; they are afraid of expressing affection in this way. This is where massage can come into its own, for it gives a perfect excuse for re-establishing contact with our fellow human beings. The lightest touch of the hand or the softest stroking movement is enough to convey sympathy, reassurance and understanding.

MASSAGING AWAY ANXIETY

Massage comforts and consoles, at the same time alleviating tensions. The world generates anxiety, every day and on every level, be it on a personal, national or international scale, from unpaid bills to a nuclear holocaust. Most of us are familiar with such troubling emotions: they make us anxious, insecure, irritable and sometimes downright depressed; however, we often remain oblivious to the disturbing physical effects of these negative states of mind.

When we are frightened or worried certain muscles contract and become tense. Everyone exhibits individual reponses but most tension settles in the neck, upper and lower back, and the hips. If tension persists, the muscle stays contracted and can become imbued with its own waste products, predominantly lactic acid. The

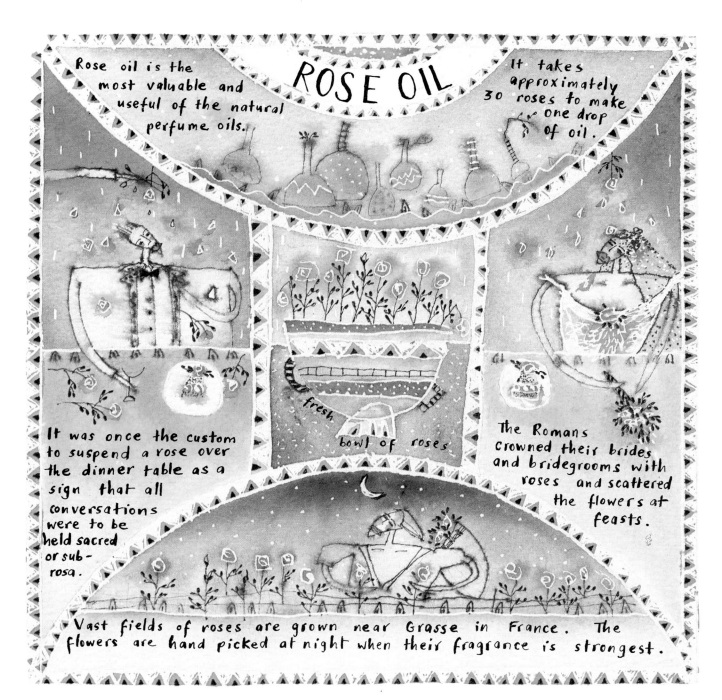

ROSE OIL

Rose oil is the most valuable and useful of the natural perfume oils.

It takes approximately 30 roses to make one drop of oil.

It was once the custom to suspend a rose over the dinner table as a sign that all conversations were to be held sacred or sub-rosa.

fresh bowl of roses

The Romans crowned their brides and bridegrooms with roses and scattered the flowers at feasts.

Vast fields of roses are grown near Grasse in France. The flowers are hand picked at night when their fragrance is strongest.

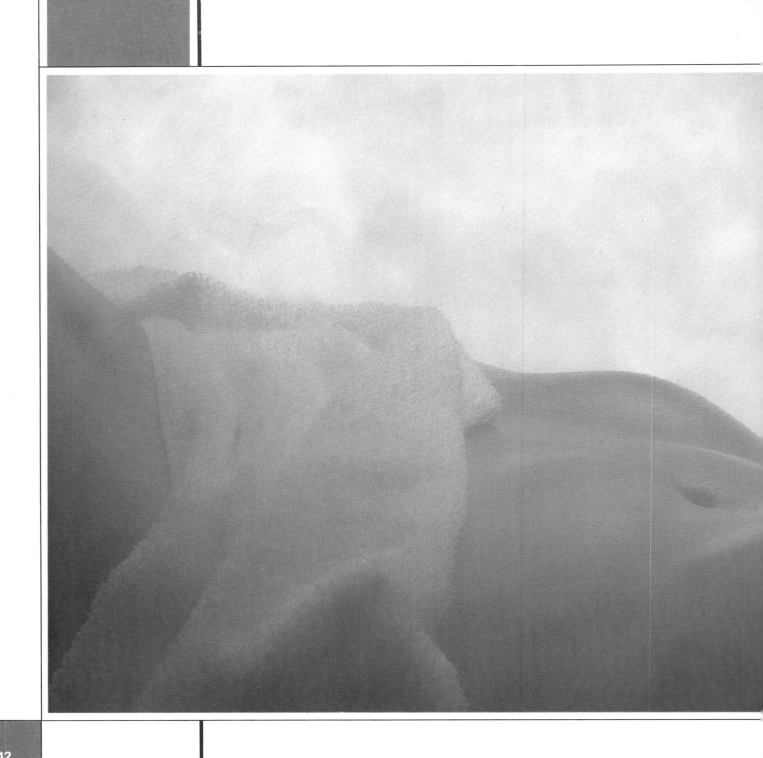

ALMOND OIL

Almond trees that bear white blossom produce bitter almonds and those with pink blossom bear sweet almonds.

Almond oil is expressed from the kernel of the sweet Almond.

almond eyes

Almond oil

almond kernels

Traditionally ripe almonds are ground into a meal and used in facial scrubs for their cleansing action.

facial scrub

In the 18th & 19th centuries Almond oil had become the main cosmetic oil and was successfully used in skin and hair preparations of many types.

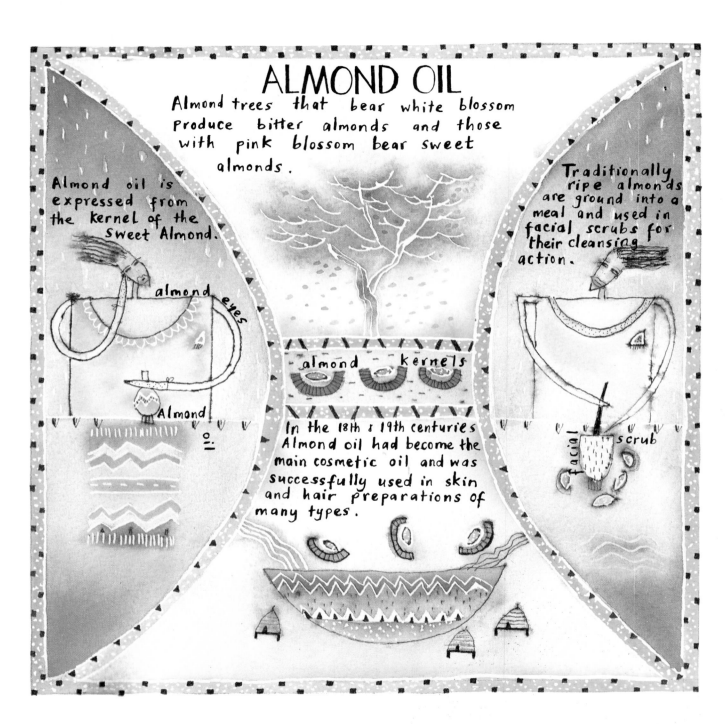

accumulated wastes prevent the muscle from relaxing and leave it stiff, sore and sometimes painful to touch. Such muscles feel like hard knots just beneath the skin surface; they are particularly likely around the shoulder blades.

By working firmly but gently on knotted muscles, wastes can be encouraged to drain away, thereby relieving stiffness and allowing the muscles to relax. There is possibly a connection between the state of mind and the state of body muscles. Wilhelm Reich, a psychologist practising at the turn of the century and a student of Sigmund Freud, thought so. He maintained that people bury anxieties and fears within their bodies in the hope of hiding them from themselves and from others. However, such emotions refuse to stay silent for long and eventually voice themselves in the form of muscular aches and pains. If you could release muscle tensions, Reich reasoned, you might possess an effective tool for relinquishing suppressed emotions. This theory could explain why people generally feel happy and relaxed after a good massage.

THE BENEFITS OF MASSAGE
By helping tense muscles to relax, massage can benefit the body in a number of ways. When a muscle is continually tensed, it becomes saturated with its own wastes, the accumulation of which makes the muscle feel sore and prevents it from working properly. Physical performance in all spheres is affected: the body works better when muscles are freed from tensions.

Ironically, wastes are also formed when a muscle is exercised. Provided that muscles are not worked excessively hard, the wastes drain away and cause no problems. However, if you push yourself beyond your limits, such wastes may stay in the muscles and are probably responsible for the "burning" sensation experienced during vigorous exercise and for the stiffness that sets in a day or so afterwards. The removal of muscle wastes, especially those produced during exercises, can be dramatically accelerated by massage; stimulating blood flow, massage encourages the delivery of nutrients and the draining away of waste products.

The ancient Greeks, who were very aware of their bodies, used massage to improve endurance and diminish fatigue more than 2000 years ago. Recent studies suggest that they knew exactly what they were doing. Normally, the recovery rate following an exercise session is about 20% after 5 minutes rest. However, after 5 minutes of massage instead of rest, muscle recovery rates are 75% or more.

MASSAGE IMPROVES HEALTHY CIRCULATION
The performance of the circulatory system is largely determined by genetic factors, though it can also be affected by diet, exercise, life-style and massage. Sluggish circulation can be improved in two ways by massage. Firstly, firm pressure applied by strokes along the arms, legs, chest and back aids the movement of blood from the heart to the extremities and back again, without increasing the heart beat rate; secondly, massage helps to relax muscles which, when tense, interfere with the free flow of blood around the body.

CHILBLAINS
People with poor circulation almost invariably suffer from chilblains in winter. Preventive measures include well-insulated gloves and thick fishermen's socks for

Fact: from the subconscious
A well-known French psychoanalyst used essential oils in the treatment of patients. He dipped cottonwool balls into oils and dangled them under the nose of his patients in an attempt to recall long-buried memories.

Fact: ancient medicine
Chinese doctors still treat a variety of illnesses, both minor and severe, by manipulating, pressing and rubbing specific areas of the body.

Opposite: Massage should be brisk, not brutal, like the movements for modelling firm clay, for brushing or rolling on paint and for kneading bread dough.

outdoor wear, and hand and foot massage for at least 5 minutes once a day, or more if possible. The Body Shop Cocoa — Butter Hand and Body Lotion is ideal for hand massage; it contains chamomile and marigold extracts to soothe sore and chapped skin, and cocoa butter which moisturises and protects the skin against harsh wintry weather and central heating.

For foot massage, use the Peppermint Foot Lotion; this also contains lubricating cocoa butter, with menthol which brings blood to the surface of the skin and warms the feet, and cooling peppermint oil to soothe itching and irritation.

DULL SKIN

Lifeless skin is frequently symptomatic of poor circulation; it does not reflect inadequate skin care, rather a lack of blood flowing through the capillaries just below the skin surface. Poor circulation probably also predisposes some women to unsightly cellulite on the hips, thighs and buttocks.

When the circulation is stimulated, the skin achieves a better texture and a more radiant appearance, because the newly forming cells receive a good supply of necessary nutrients; cellulite can then be reduced and, more significantly, prevented.

MASSAGE, THE ULTIMATE CLEANSER

The lymphatic system plays a vital role in determining how well we look and feel. All cells in the body are bathed in a tissue fluid which diffuses from the blood capillaries; while some of the fluid returns to the capillaries, the remainder, which is known as lymph, picks up metabolic wastes, dead cells, bacteria and other undesirable particles and drains into thin-walled lymphatic vessels. These form a network in the body, channelling lymph from the tissues to the heart. At intervals throughout the network, lymph is filtered through small tissue swellings known as lymph nodes where harmful bacteria and viruses are ingested by the protective white blood cells. The major lymph nodes are found in the neck, the armpits, the groin and at the backs of the knees. Unlike blood, which is pumped around the body by the heart, movement of the lymph depends partly on compression by the muscles in the arms and legs and partly on the suction created with every breath. At the onset of an infection, the lymph nodes produce antibodies as a defence, and the nodes sometimes swell and become painful.

Puffy-looking skin and muscles, whose distinct outlines have become blurred, are commonly accompanied by a stagnating lymphatic system when metabolic wastes and other toxins are not being efficiently removed from the tissues.

Massage effectively encourages lymphatic draingage, cleansing the body of unwanted substances and defining body contours. Gentle strokes mimic the pumping action of the muscles to speed the flow of lymph through the body. **Work towards the heart,** using long sweeping movements from the fingers along the arms towards the nodes in the armpits, then down over the chest. Work down the neck, over and across the shoulders and down towards the heart. Finally, work from the toes up the legs, over the knees and towards the groin area. The lymphatic system works hand in hand with the liver and kidneys, organs responsible for the elimination of body wastes; speeding the flow of blood to these organs, massage helps them to perform their functions more efficiently.

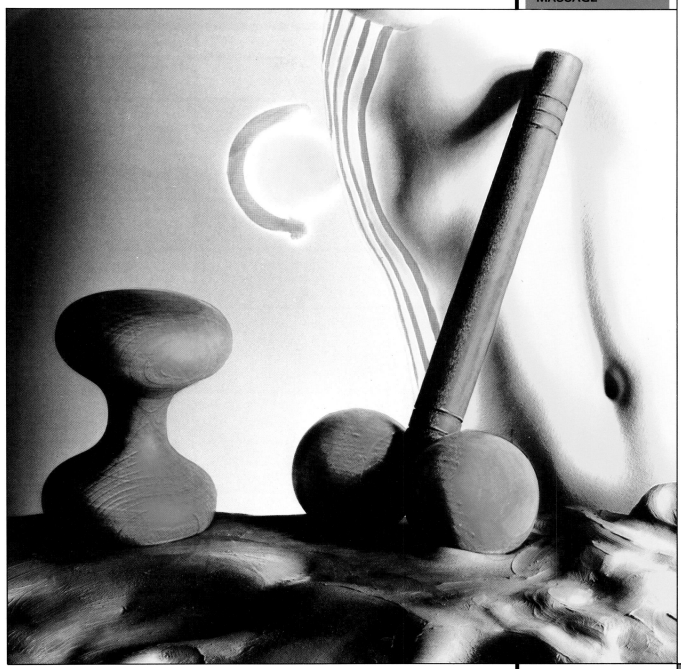

MASSAGE TOOLS AND EQUIPMENT

TOOL	DESCRIPTION	USAGE	ADVANTAGES
BACK RUB	Wooden implement, of Chinese design	Rubbing up and down spine over pressure points	Improves circulation; gives relief from muscle tension
BODY BUDDY	Rubber mitt, one side with small rubber bristles, the other with rounded nodules	Use for massage in bath or shower, bristle side on body, legs and arms, the other side on thighs, buttocks and hips	Promotes blood flow through capillaries close to skin surface; tones fleshy areas
BODY TONER	Solid beech ridged-roller	Use on thighs, calfs and bottom of feet	Stimulates circulation; encourages mobilization of fatty deposits
CONTOUR CARESSER	Series of beechwood wheels in macramé frame; handles at both ends	Rub and roll over back and shoulders, buttocks and back of thighs	Relaxes shoulder and back muscles; tones thighs and buttocks
FOOTSIE ROLLER	Wooden roller, sculpted for foot massage	In sitting position, place feet on roller and roll it forwards and backwards over the soles, with steady pressure	Ideal for warming up feet before strenuous exercise and for cooling them down afterwards
MASSAGE BAND	Woven coarse hemp	Back massage	Sloughs away dead skin cells; stimulates circulation
MINI-MASSEUR	Wooden massage roller	Roll and rub over leg, arm and shoulder muscles	Relaxes tense muscles, eases fatigue
SCALP MASSAGER	Small round plastic disc covered with fine plastic bristles	Work thoroughly over entire scalp, preferably just before a shampoo	Stimulates circulation; improves hair growth
SISAL BODY BRUSH	Pure sisal fibres, plastic-backed hand brush with strap	Ideal for wet or dry body massage	Sloughs off dead skin cells, stimulates circulation and lymphatic drainage; thought to promote the elimination of wastes through the skin

MASSAGE, THE NATURAL PAINKILLER

The instinctive reaction to pain is to rub the affected area, and with good reason. Research into pain control has revealed that rubbing is one of the body's natural pain-blocking processes. According to the *Gate Control Theory*, proposed by Professors Ronald Melzack and Patrick Wall, rubbing stimulates touch receptors found abundantly in the skin. They in turn send impulses to the brain, passing first through a "gate" in the spinal chord; touch impulses travel faster than pain, and by the time this arrives at the gate, it has already closed.

Rubbing prevents pain information from reaching the brain and is helpful for relieving stiff necks, backaches, fractures, period pains and childbirth.

BACK PAIN

Four out of five adults will suffer from backache at some point in their lives. It is estimated that every year 2 million people in Britain visit their doctors with back complaints, with a subsequent loss of some 13 million working days. Massage is one of the most effective means of preventing and relieving back pain which in the majority of cases is caused by chronic muscle tension.

Most muscle tension has developed over a number of years; it rarely occurs overnight but is the result of poor posture. Sitting hunched over a typewriter or desk puts tremendous strain on certain muscles in the neck and upper back; other jobs, and sport activities, that force the body into unnatural positions also create muscular tensions. By repeated misuse of the body, certain muscles become so tense that circulation is shut off and as wastes are not being removed, the muscles go into spasms. Many people lead a sedentary life and the back muscles are those most affected and abused. Problems arise from crystals formed in the constricted area, causing muscle fibres to adhere and cement the tension. The back muscles are attached to the vertebrae in the spinal column, and if they are very tense they can pull the spine out of line, a common cause of back pain.

A good massage can disperse the crystals, restoring movement to the muscles and preventing back pain. Qualified remedial masseurs with a good knowledge of physiology can relieve chronic back pain. **This should never be attempted by the amateur.** It is also within the capabilities of qualified masseurs to help injuries, such as sprains, heal more quickly, and – provided they are caught in their early stages – to prevent conditions like arthritis and bursitis from getting any worse.

Important: do not try to treat chronic backache with ordinary massage. In some instances it may well make matters worse.

MASSAGE STROKES

A typical Swedish massage employs several techniques which aim to soothe tension and promote relaxation, boost blood and lymph circulation, improve muscle tone and flexibility of the joints, and to revive flagging energy levels.

EFFLEURAGE

A long stroking movement which introduces the sensation of touch to the skin. It warms and relaxes, while stimulating the blood circulation and lymph flow throughout the body. Using both hands, glide over the skin applying a constant, even pressure on every part of the body. Slow gentle movements.

Warning: under pressure
In some countries, masseurs walk up and down the spine in order to apply extra pressure. It probably wouldn't go down well if you suggested this to your partner. You could compromise by using elbows and knuckles if your thumbs and fingers become tired.

Tip: balm for pains
Cool Eucalyptus Oil soothes muscular aches, among other things; a back rub with Tangerine Oil, ideal for children and pregnant mums, reduces anxiety.

Fact: power points
The concept of pressure-point massage was introduced to Japan by Buddhist monks in the 6th century. Today, the Nippon Shiatsu School boasts some 20,000 graduates.

Opposite: *In tapotment the massage strokes on back and legs are similar to the rapid taps of drumsticks and the soft swish of a brush.*

PETRISSAGE

This is the rhythmic lifting, squeezing and rolling of muscles with the hands. It pumps nutrients through the muscles and drains away wastes while acting on the deeper blood and lymph vessels. Take hold of the flesh between thumb and fingers and pull it away from the bone, squeezing as if kneading a piece of dough. Use on soft parts of the body as well as on the muscles. Firm movements.

FRICTION

A rapid oscillating movement which helps to disperse crystals that "glue" muscle fibres together. It increases the blood supply to internal organs. A useful stroke for stiff joints. Place the palms of the hands on the particular area of the body and with even pressure rub them back and forth energetically. Firm movements.

TAPOTMENT

Also known as percussion, this is the cupping, slapping, hacking and chopping motions of the hands usually associated with massage. Tapotment works to stimulate or sedate the nerves, depending on how long it is performed. It also improves muscle tone and helps to firm sagging skin. Use on the back and along the backs of the legs. Properly performed, with the wrists loose and flexible, the movements should be invigorating, never painful. Fast movements.

PUTTING ON THE PRESSURE

Pressure applied to specific points on the body forms the basis for therapies like acupressure, shiatsu, touch for health, and reflexology. According to ancient Chinese medical lore, numerous pathways along which energy flows, run through the body. Unlike the circulatory and lymphatic systems the energy pathways or meridians cannot be seen, which for some sceptics is sufficient to doubt their existence. However, modern electronic equipment has been able to trace energy pathways that correspond to the Chinese acupuncture meridians.

A total of 59 meridians are used in traditional Chinese acupuncture, and it is thought that each meridian is associated with a particular organ or bodily function. In a healthy, balanced condition, energy flows smoothly along the meridians, supplying and maintaining all parts of the body. However, if the body is weakened by illness, emotional stress, injury or an immoderate life-style, the energy flow can become blocked at certain points, resulting in an excess in some areas and a deficiency in others. When this happens we become prone to emotional upsets, such as moodiness and depression, and to physical ailments like upset stomachs, pre-menstrual tension and headaches.

Various points along the meridians act like amplifiers, passing energy from one point to another. These are the points into which the acupuncturists stick tiny needles; it is also possible to remove the blockage and restore a balanced energy flow along the meridian by applying firm finger pressure to the appropriate points.

SHIATSU

This is the Japanese interpretation of Chinese acupuncture; it also incorporates the principles of other massage techniques. Most Shiatsu is based on 12 basic Chinese acupuncture meridians; the energy is referred to as *ki*, and the pressure points, of

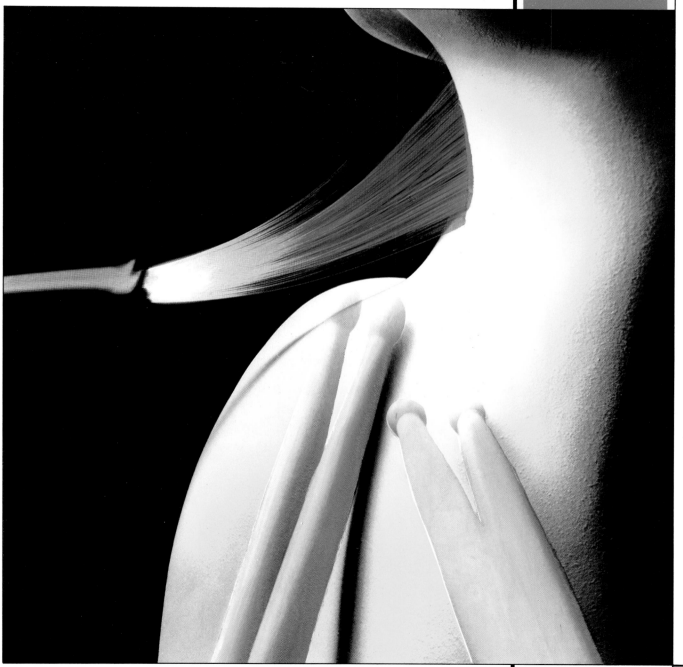

Tip: Shiatsu for feet
Relieve tired feet by pressing the toes, then the upper tendons towards the ankles. Next, work the soles, the arches, around the ankles, and finally the Achilles heel.

which there are some 365 over the entire body surface, are called *tsubos*. The Japanese Ministry of Health and Welfare states that Shiatsu therapy can "correct internal malfunctioning, promote health and treat specific diseases". In the West, Shiatsu is one of the lesser known therapies, but interest is growing among professional masseurs in its therapeutic potentials.

In order to treat a specific problem by working the pressure points a tremendous knowledge of the meridians and their roles, as well as a good understanding of the way the human body works, are obviously essential, but there is no reason why you should not extend your massage by working various pressure points.

The points easiest to locate lie on either side of the entire length of the spine, along the so-called bladder meridian. Using the "soles" or pads of the thumbs, not the tips, apply firm pressure to the point and hold it for 3-10 seconds before releasing. You will know when you have found a pressure point or *tsubo* because it will feel slightly tender. Starting at the top of the spine and working downwards, touch on the points between the shoulder blades, to stimulate circulation and help to relieve anxiety, distress and insomnia. The points in the middle-back region are concerned with digestion, those in the lumbar region (lower back) influence the kidneys and help to control water retention. Working down the spine stimulates the spinal nerves which supply all the internal organs, and almost every point on the back influences the supply of energy to the other meridians.

Other pressure points, which should be easy to find, run across the tops of the

Pressure points *on the face relate to specific actions: those at the temples promote calmness, those below the eyebrows relieve fatigue, and those by the bridge of the nose and by the nostrils ease congestion. Pressure on the cheek points reduces swelling, and on the jaw bones improves lymph flow.*

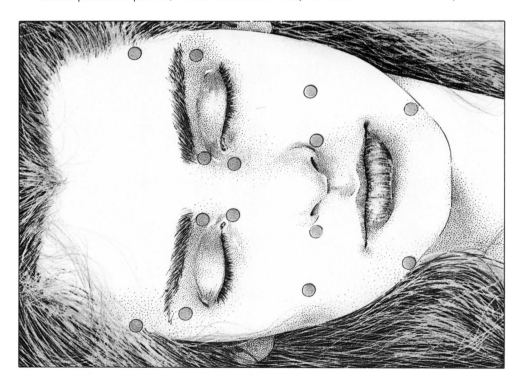

shoulders; working these helps to relieve stress and tensions and soothes head-aches and colds. Moving down to the hips, apply pressure to points close to the "sacral dips" or dimples on either side of the spine; this is especially soothing and relaxing for women, and helps to relieve period pains. The bladder meridian continues down the back of the legs. Pressing the points at the back of the knees can relieve emotional strain and release tension in the knees.

Six different meridians run the length of the arms. By working the points at the top of the arm and in the crease of the elbow, you can encourage the elimination of body wastes, which is helpful for treating blemished skins, and also improves circulation, respiration and digestion.

REFLEXOLOGY

The precise origins are unknown. It is a type of pressure-point massage for the hands and feet which probably evolved from a massage technique practised thousands of years ago in China. For the purposes of reflexology, the body is divided into ten different zones, five on each half of the body. Each toe represents a zone or energy channel which travels longitudinally up the body to the head and extends to the hands, or rather the fingers and thumb. Any organ, gland or part of the body occurring within a particular zone will have its reflex in the corresponding zone of the head and foot. If an area of the hand or foot feels particularly tender, the pain, to a trained reflexologist, will indicate tension or congestion in some part of the body which lies within the same zone.

In order that treatment can be specific, scaled-down maps of the body appear on the bottom of our feet and palms of our hands. The theory is that by working a point on the hand or the foot that corresponds to a certain part of the body, such as the eye, liver or stomach, its function can be affected. This sounds feasible, for the nerves that pass through the body's organs do end in the hands and feet, and crystalline deposits of uric acid and calcium often form at the nerve endings, preventing the nerves from functioning efficiently. Pressure applied to the reflex points helps to dissolve these crystals which are absorbed back into the bloodsteam and eliminated in the normal way. The breakdown and dispersal or these crystalline deposits benefit both the particular nerves and the organs they innervate within the zone; at the same time circulation is improved and muscles toned up, resulting in transferred tension relief throughout the body.

A thorough hand and foot massage is a marvellous way of reviving anyone who is tired or jaded. Such massage will also work to release congestion in the body resulting from heavy stress, bad diet, lack of sleep, an alcoholic evening, etc. Reflexologists claim that they can treat ailing organs and glands by working the feet and hands, and at the same time discover which parts of the body are not functioning as efficiently as they might.

A special kind of thumb pressure is used professionally to work the reflex points. It involves digging the tip of the thumb into the relevant area, while supporting the rest of the hand or foot with the fingers and working across the area like a caterpillar, alternately bending and straightening the thumb.

You can use reflexology as an antidote for many everyday problems. It is not necessary to incorporate it in a full body massage; simply work the particular reflex points for 30 seconds or so, two or three times a day or whenever the need arises.

Tip: childbirth
Reflexology can be beneficial at childbirth. By working the relevant points, a trained therapist can strengthen weak contractions, thereby speeding up the delivery of the baby. It may also be used to induce labour in women who are overdue – providing a natural alternative to drugs.

Tip: reflexology into massage
The foot is sensitive to touch. After pouring oil into your hands, and before beginning the massage, hold the left foot firmly, press for about 20 seconds along the underneath area and upper surface. This induces a feeling of relaxation.

OFFICE HEADACHES

Work over the pad of the thumb (from the knuckle joint to the tip), concentrating on the area closest to the forefinger which is confusingly known as the outside. Treat both hands.

MID-AFTERNOON FATIGUE

This can be alleviated by stimulating the adrenal glands. To locate the appropriate point, trace a straight line across the palm beginning from the point at which the thumb joins the hand. Drop another imaginary line from the join of the first and second finger. Where these lines meet you will find the adrenals. Treat both hands.

INSOMNIA

If you are unable to sleep because of tension or racing thoughts, or have trouble unwinding, it may help to work the solar plexus reflex point, which can be found at the centre of the palm. Press the point for ½-1 minute. Treat both hands.

PERIOD PAINS

Two points on the feet can be worked in order to relieve period pains. They correspond to the uterus and the ovaries; the reflex point for the ovaries is on the outside of each foot, just below and to the back of the ankle bone. The uterus point lies on the inside of each foot, almost directly opposite the ovary reflex points. The uterus can also be reached by pressing on each side of the Achilles tendon, the hard ligament at the back of the ankle.

INDIGESTION

A meal consumed too quickly can cause gas to build up in the colon. This puts pressure on the spleen, diaphragm and heart, often resulting in bloating and heartburn. The colon, heart and spleen all lie in the zone corresponding to a band running along the outside of the left foot. Start from the little toe and work along the bottom of the foot towards the heel.

WORKAHOLICS' BACKACHE

At the end of a working day spent over a typewriter or desk, the chances are that the back will ache. Treat the spinal area whose reflex points run up the inside of each foot; begin from the big toe and work along the foot towards the heel.

COLDS IN THE HEAD

Perhaps the most unpleasant aspect of a cold is congestion of the sinuses; it brings a dull aching headache clouding the thinking ability. Catarrh can be encouraged to drain from the tissues by working the sinus reflex points. They are found on the pads of the toes except the big toes.

CREATING THE ATMOSPHERE

For a massage to be truly beneficial, it should take place in comfortable, relaxing conditions. Choose a room free from draughts, because chilly gusts will immediately make the muscles contract, and ensure that the room is properly warmed up in advance; the ideal temperature for a massage is supposed to be about 21°C. If you are giving a full body massage with oil, the person will be naked; keep a blanket handy to cover up the parts of the body you are not working on. Keep the lighting soft; daylight is fine, providing it is filtered, but candlelight is more restful.

The room can be scented with fresh flowers or potpourri; it is not essential and neither is music, though a gentle rhythmic piece may help you to give a flowing massage, fill the silence and relax the other person. The right surface for a massage is of particular importance. Special tables which bring the person to be massaged up to waist level are ideal, but few of us possess that type of equipment; the next best thing is the floor. If the room is carpeted, a sleeping bag covered with a couple of rugs or blankets will do, otherwise use a thick foam mat. Never massage someone on a bed or matress; it cannot give the support necessary for the strokes to be effective. Cover the massage surface with a sheet to catch any splashes of oil.

While you massage on the front of the body, place a cushion or small pillow under the head of the "patient", to help release tension in the neck, and another under the knees. For a back massage, remove the pillow under the head.

MASSAGE OILS

Oil lubricates the skin and makes stroking and kneading movements smooth and comfortable. The most suitable oil is light and easily absorbed so that when the excess is tissued off, the skin feels soft and supple, not unpleasantly sticky. The Body Shop Massage Oil is based on soya oil which is light in texture, pale yellow in colour and odourless; scent with aromatherapy oil or perfume.

Sweet Almond Oil is also excellent; it is slightly heavier, and contains significant quantities of vitamins E and F which help to feed the skin. It is ideal for hand massage because rubbed into the cuticles the oil helps to strengthen the growing nails.

Apricot Kernel Oil, a lightweight emollient oil, contains vitamin A which maintains healthy skin and surface tissues; it is particularly good for softening hard, rough skin.

Pressure points on the hands are easily located and worked for half a minute at a time: for headaches and neck pains, press the pads on the thumbs; relieve a cold in the head by working the reflex points on the fingers. Counteract fatigue by stimulating the adrenal glands corresponding to the point in the palm nearest the thumb. Conversely, you can overcome insomnia by working the solar plexus point in the centre of the palm.

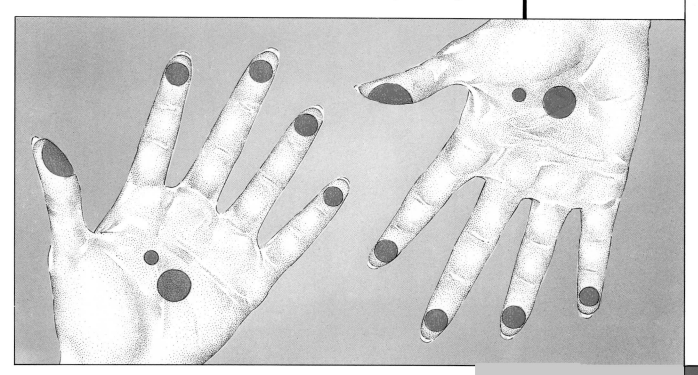

Warning: switch-off
Massage should be restful, for you and your friend. Before you start, forget any worries and empty your mind of mundane thoughts so that you can concentrate on the treatment you are giving.

Tip: coming up for air
During massage, concentrate on breathing regularly, more slowly and deeply than normally. It will help to establish a good massage rhythm and prevent you from tiring too quickly.

Antidote *to menstrual pains: work the reflex points for the ovaries on the outside of each foot, just below and behind the ankle (top). The uterus can be activated by the corresponding points on the inside of each foot, or by pressing either side of the Achilles tendon.*

Before use, warm the oil slightly by placing the bottle in a bowl of hot water for a couple of minutes. Pour about a teaspoon of oil into the hand and stroke it over the body; as you move from one area of the body to another, apply a little more oil.

Some people do not like the feel of oil on their skin. The Body Shop Rich Massage Lotion is a rich lotion with the comforting aroma of vanilla; it is extremely lubricating and allows you to massage for up to half and hour before reapplication. It is suitable for all skin types and particularly good for skin dehydrated by over-exposure to sun and sea. The lotion is also useful for massaging a stiff leg muscle or sore shoulder; it is quickly absorbed and leaves no traces of grease on your clothes.

GIVING A MASSAGE

Before you start a massage, you should familiarize yourself with the sequence of movements. Most books on massage include a step-by-step guide to giving a body massage. Unless you have a photographic memory, you will work in fits and starts, checking the text. Nothing spoils a massage more than a break of contact for every touch is a part of the experience.

In order to give a good massage you must establish and maintain a steady rhythm throughout, and move swiftly, almost imperceptibly from one part of the body to another. Once you have grasped the basic massage techniques, follow your intuition. First try out the various strokes on yourself to discover what feels best where, then try them on a friend and ask for an honest opinion.

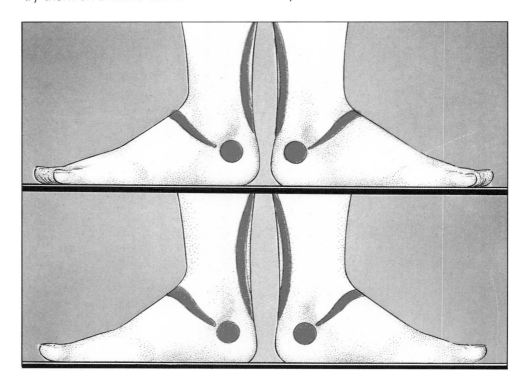

BASIC MASSAGE SEQUENCE

Begin with the back:
* Start from the buttocks and stroke lightly up the back. As the skin warms up, apply firmer pressure.
* Follow with friction, then petrissage. There is little flesh on the back, but you can squeeze and knead the shoulders, hips and buttocks.
* Work the pressure points (see reflexology) down the spine and over the shoulders and hips.
* Follow with tapotment; be gentle on the back, energetic over the buttocks.
* Finish with effleurage.

THE LEGS

Massage and finish the back of one leg at a time:
* Stroke lightly down the leg and firmly back up to the buttocks to encourage the flow of blood and lymph.
* Use friction on the ankle joint and over the back of the knee.
* The pressure points can be worked now if desired.
* Follow with petrissage and tapotment, and end with stroking down to the foot.
* Work over the whole foot with firm circling thumb movements. Concentrate on the soles where the reflex points lie and try to break down any gritty crystalline deposits.
* Rub the foot briskly.
* Stroke up the leg, over the back to the shoulders, let your hands rest here for a moment, then ask the person to roll over.

THE ARMS

Massage one arm at a time:
* Holding the "patient's" hand in your left (or right) hand, stroke lightly from the shoulder to the wrist, then firmly back up to the shoulder, first on the outside, then on the inside of the arm.
* Let go of the arm and follow with petrissage, working up the arm from the wrist. Be gentle on thinly fleshed, sensitive areas, and use both hands to squeeze and knead the flesh of the upper arm.
* Work the pressure points if you like.
* Stroke down the arm and over the hand.

* Massage the hand in the same way as the foot, with particular attention to the palms, using firm circling movements with the thumb. Grasp each finger between thumb and forefinger and pull from the joint to the finger tip, working the knuckles as you stroke over them.
* Stroke the whole hand several times.

THE CHEST AND STOMACH

* Stroke down the neck, then out towards the shoulders. Move from the neck down over the collar bone to the chest, lightly at first, followed by firmer strokes.
* Follow with friction over the entire chest area if you are very familiar with your friend; otherwise skip the chest and stroke lightly down over the ribs towards the stomach.
* Using the palm of one hand stroke firmly over the abdomen in a clockwise direction several times.
* Follow with petrissage; knead and squeeze the flesh round the waist and hips.
* Stroke slowly and firmly from the stomach up the rib cage; glide back down and repeat several times.
* Finish by gently stroking the whole area.
* Massage the front of the legs in the same way as you did the back of them.

THE HEAD

The best position for a head massage is sitting on a chair, with your friend on the floor in front of you, leaning back against your knees. Wash your hands and make sure they are free from all traces of oil before you begin.
* Stroke lightly from the forehead, over the top of the head and down to the neck. Repeat, starting from the temple and stroking over the ears. Follow with firmer stroking movements.
* Using thumbs and fingertips, work in firm circular movements over the entire surface of the head, concentrating on the top of the skull, round the ears and the top of the neck where tension often builds up.
* Hold the head firmly between both hands and gently tilt it forwards and backwards, then from side to side.
* Finish by stroking the whole head lightly with the fingertips.

Tip: beautiful thoughts
The person you are massaging may find it difficult to relax. Tell her to think of something pleasant, like a white sandy beach lapped with turquoise-blue waves, or imagine the warm sun on her back and the touch of a soft summer breeze.

Tip: on feet
Massage the feet with moistened coarse salt, baking soda or avocado flesh before soaking them with water.

Tip: foot exercise
Massage the feet by wearing socks with a handful of dried peas. It is as effective as walking on pebbles.

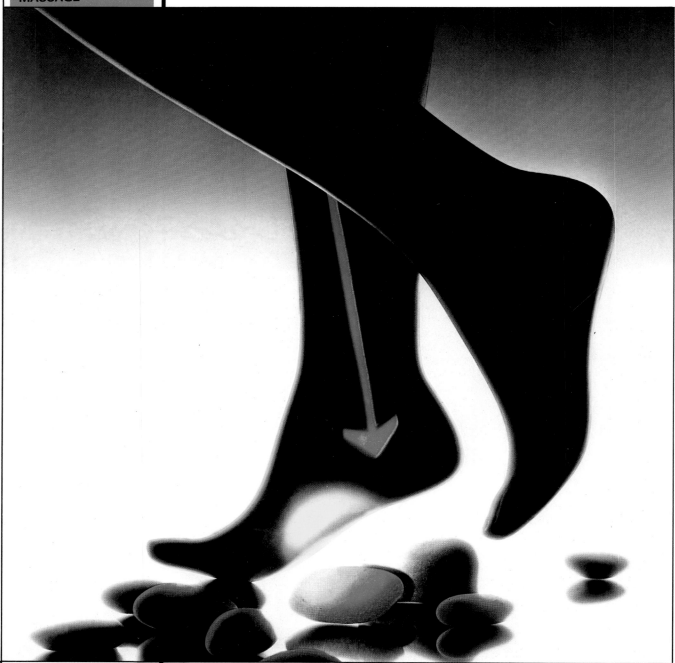

A head massage is marvellous for getting somebody who is very tense to relax quickly. It does not involve removal of a single item of clothing, and oil is not necessary. You can easily give yourself a head massage: when you shampoo your hair, take a few extra minutes to massage the scalp thoroughly; it helps to relax tense muscles, stimulates circulation and encourages nutrients to the follicles.

Treat yourself or a friend to a massage with Body Shop Aromatherapy Scalp Oil. This is a light blend of almond and wheatgerm oil, with essential oils including lavender for hair growth, juniper to strengthen skin and scalp tissues, rosemary to encourage the flow of blood through the scalp tissues and to act as a dandruff cleanser, and cypress to soothe the scalp. The oil is excellent for scalp massage in general and is particularly helpful for sufferers from dandruff, dry, itchy scalp and hair loss. Once a week, massage the oil into the scalp, leave it on for half an hour, then wash with Orange Spice Shampoo.

DO-IT-YOURSELF MASSAGE
Most people think of massage as something that is done by others instead of a do-it-yourself performance. It is naturally more relaxing to lie back and let someone else do the hard worik, but we can still benefit greatly from massaging ourselves. There are certain areas such as the back which it is difficult to work properly, though some of the massage tools come in handy. In order to reap the full benefits of massage it must be done regularly, like cleaning the teeth, and unless you have a generous partner or friend, that means doing it yourself. Try to spare half an hour extra and include massage in your daily routine.

One of the best times to fit in massage is during a shower or a bath. Instead of oil to lubricate the skin, use a fast-foaming liquid soap to reduce the friction between your hands and the skin. Body Shop's Herbal Body Shampoo and Strawberry Body Shampoo are ideal. Use a Skin Towel or Skin Sponge for effleurage; they are made of mildly abrasive Japanese fibres which slough away dead cells.

After bathing, the skin is warm and the muscles relaxed; this is a perfect time to indulge in petrissage, friction and tapotment, even while watching television. There are other occasions when massage is, if not essential, beneficial and relaxing:

* after a particularly stressful day; it releases tension before this has a chance to manifest itself in the muscles.
* when you are utterly exhausted; it will cleanse the body of the chemicals that cause fatigue; a quick massage is a better and safer pick-me-up than a cup of black coffee or a stiff drink.

* whenever the skin looks puffy; this is a sign that the lymphatic system needs a little boost.
* after a day spent sitting in an aeroplane, train or the office. It can substitute for the exercise you missed, helping to stimulate the flow of blood and lymph and leave you feeling refreshed and revitalized.

FACIAL MASSAGE
The muscles which cover the face are largely responsible for its smooth contours and for the expressions that mirror our emotions. Like any other muscles, the facial muscles are subject to tension; with constant anxiety, frown or worry lines become indelibly etched, but a massage to relax contracted muscles can be as effective as a long, lazy holiday. It can also improve the tone of weak, underused muscles, such as those round the jawline, and help to preserve the youthful contours of the face.

Warning: off colour?
Never attempt to massage someone else if you are about to go down with a cold or other illness. Your energy levels are bound to be low, and you may worsen matters by using up your reserves on somebody else.

Tip: self knowledge
Giving yourself a massage is the ideal way of reaching a better understanding of your body. When you can translate body signals into physical and mental needs, you can protect yourself against much illness, pain and emotional trauma.

Opposite: *Foot massage does more than exercise the feet, for the benefits show in relaxed face muscles, a straight back, good posture and springy gait. Scrunch barefoot on smooth pebbles or marbles.*

Rhythmic stroking movements speed the flow of blood and lymph through the tissues; a good facial massage can reduce puffiness round the eyes and cheeks and leave the skin looking refreshed and glowing. Firm finger-pressure applied for 3-5 seconds to the pressure points on the face can help banish fatigue, relieve sinus congestion, alleviate headaches, lift the spirits and erase fine lines.

Before beginning a massage cleanse the face thoroughly. Remove all traces of make-up and follow with a facial sauna. Fill the basin or sink with scalding hot water, lean over it, your head covered with a towel to seal in the steam. Remain like that for 5 minutes. If you suffer, even slightly, from broken veins, leave this step out.

After steaming, pat the face dry with a towel or paper tissue. The skin will now be warm and moist, the facial muscles beginning to relax and primed for massage. Pour a teaspoon of the chosen oil into your hands and apply to the skin; use more oil as soon as the skin feels in need of lubrication.

MASSAGE MOVEMENTS

1. With the fingertips stroke up from the neck and circle out over the cheeks. Then sweep from the centre of the forehead out to the temples. Hold the pressure points at the temples with the tips of the second fingers to induce tranquility.
2. Place forefinger and middle finger flat against the forehead and make rapid scissoring movements. Then stroke from the forehead out to the temples.
3. Hold the pressure point at the inside of the eye socket, at the beginning of the eyebrow, to ease fatigue. Sweep in a semi-circle out over the eyebrow, and hold the pressure point in the hollow outside the eye socket, at the end of the eyebrow.
4. Sweep in a semi-circle back under the eye. Repeat 3 and 4 several times.
5. With the first three fingers of each hand roll up under the jawline, the hands moving simultaneously to tone slack muscles.
6. Pinch round the jawline with thumb and forefinger, starting at the chin and working out towards the ears. This helps to ward off a double chin.
7. Hold the pressure points midway along the jaw bones to improve lymph flow.
8. Apply pressure to points either side of the bridge of the nose, close to the inside of the eyes. Then work in small rotating movements down along each side of the nose. Hold the point at the outer edge of each nostril to ease nasal congestion.
9. Make small rotating movements with fingertips from the corners of the mouth, out over the cheeks to the ears. Press pressure points under the cheeks to reduce swelling.
10. Finally stroke down the neck from chin to shoulder, alternating one hand with the other, to aid lymphatic drainage.

A complete facial massage takes time. If you cannot afford that, try a mini facial massage when you cleanse your face or apply moisturiser. It will pep up the complexion first thing in the morning and help you to unwind at night.

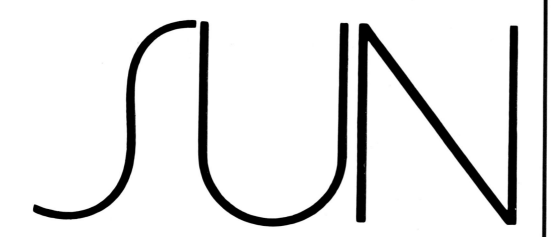

SUN

SUN ON THE SKIN

SUN ON THE FACE

SUN ON THE BODY

SUN ON THE HAIR

AFTER SUN

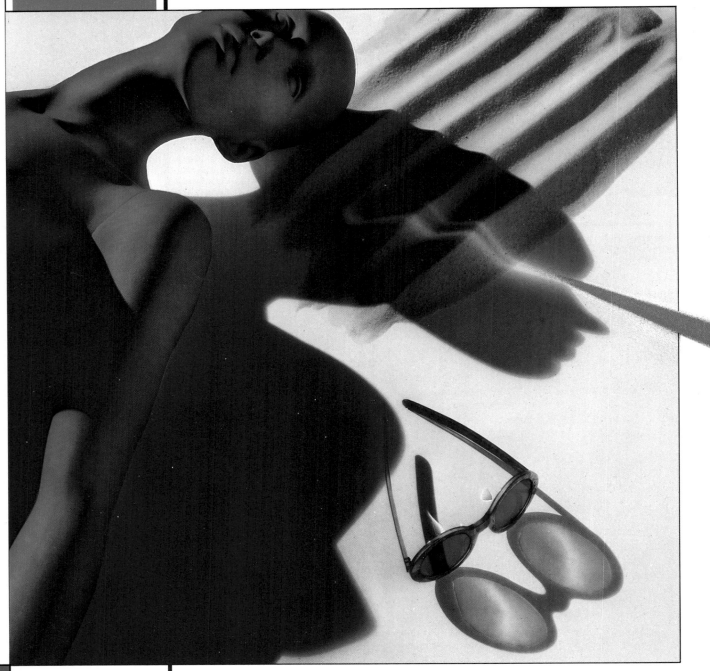

SUN ON THE SKIN

THINK OF THE POSITIVE APPEAL OF PALE SKIN: BEFORE THE SECOND World War no one considered the *deliberate* act of burning the skin to be essential to beauty. The pioneers trekking across the American continent were concerned to protect their skin against the fierce sun; the Victorians considered sunburnt skin as typical of peasants, and freckles as the worst possible blemish a girl could suffer. Anxious mamas made sure their daughters never went outside without their parasols. Today, dermatologists would agree with the Victorians, if for different reasons.

Pale hands and faces are becoming the vogue as they were in Victorian days, and cosmetic companies produce paler shades of foundations and powders. The reasons for this trend are easy to understand as the number of admissions to dermatologists' clinics for sun-related skin damage, including cancer, escalates alarmingly. In addition to this, the sun works unseen havoc on the lower levels of the skin, and while brown may be beautiful to look at, the beauty is literally only skin-deep.

THE DANGERS OF A SUNTAN

Research has revealed that the sun's ultraviolet rays, previously thought to be "harmless" tanning rays, penetrate to the lower levels of the epidermis to accelerate the ageing process. **Too much sun and too little protection is bad for you:** it leads irrevocably to ageing of the skin, with wrinkles, brown patches and loss of elasticity.

As most people in the UK spend only a few weeks every year grilling under strong sun, the acquisition of a tan is not necessarily the road to dermatological ruin, but you should be aware of the dangers in exposing the skin to the rays of the sun, and how you can minimize those dangers while still acquiring an attractive colour.

SKIN AND ITS FUNCTIONS

The skin is one of the body's largest organs and receives about one third of the blood supply. In some places, such as the soles of the feet, the palms of the hands and the upper back, it is quite thick, while in others it is very thin – probably thinnest on the eyelids, where it is only about 0.5mm thick. The average adult has 16.000 sq cm of skin, and it is a surprisingly busy canvas. In each square centimetre there are approximately 10 hairs, 100 sweat glands, one metre of blood vessels, 15 sebaceous glands and 4 metres of nerves, with 3000 sensory cells at the end of nerve fibres to record pain, pressure, heat and cold.

The skin's most important function is to protect the body. It is our defence against bacteria, harmful chemicals and other hazards; it also prevents us from losing too much water. It helps to regulate body temperature and is an important part of the way we assess our environment through the sensory cells.

Protection and care of the skin is more than a beauty issue. Any influence, such as the sun, which causes the skin to react and change must be seriously considered.

Warning: Slip, Slop, Slap
In Australia, where people spend a lot of time outdoors, many women in their early thirties look ten years older than their age, and the incidence of fatal skin cancers (malignant melanomas) has reached alarming proportions. A TV commercial, mounted by the Australian Government Health Department, advises:
Slip on a shirt
Slop on sunscreen
Slap on a hat

Opposite: *Ultraviolet rays may cause eye strain, and tunnel vision in extreme cases. Keep the head in the shade while sunbathing and wear sun glasses to prevent wrinkles round the eyes.*

Danger
The short UVB rays are the ones to avoid, especially when they are directly overhead: on top of a mountain where the thin air allows them to burn more fiercely; and between 11 in the morning and 3 in the afternoon.

WHAT THE SUN DOES TO SKIN

The sun emits three kinds of rays relevant to tanning: Ultraviolet A (UVA), Ultraviolet B (UVB) and Ultraviolet C (UVC). The rest of the sun's rays are visible light and infrared – if you could see the whole spectrum it would look like a rainbow. By the time sunlight reaches the earth, the UVC rays, which are potentially the most dangerous, have been absorbed or deflected by the protective upper atmosphere. Of the two rays that reach our skin the UVA are the longer tanning rays, and the UVB the shorter, burning rays. Only the ultraviolet rays have the correct wavelength to actually penetrate the skin and affect the lower levels; the rest of the light spectrum is harmless and bounces off. One of the skin's functions is to protect internal organs from possible external dangers, and the skin cells recognize UV rays as aliens – deadly enemies to be opposed at all costs.

When both sets of UV rays hit our skin the blood capillaries near the surface increase their permeability and the skin turns bright red – a phenomenon known to the medical profession as erythema and to the holidaymaker as agony. The UV rays also cause the formation of substances called "free radicals" which run riot through the skin cells, damaging the DNA, the collagen and the elastin, all elements essential to the elasticity and renewal process of the skin. It is this aspect of suntanning that scientists believe causes the skin to age faster.

The UVB rays burn far more than they tan, and it is unnecessary to "burn" at all in order to achieve a good tan. If you burn too much you will merely peel off whatever

Sunburn and melanin
are interrelated. Like effervescent bubbles rising to the surface of aerated water in a glass (left), so melanin rushes from the lower layers when the surface skin begins to burn. As part of its defence strategem, melanin tries to protect the skin by tanning it. It will do so more painlessly if it is allowed to follow its steady progression up through the skin, rather like the lazy swirls in a glass shaded from the sun (right).

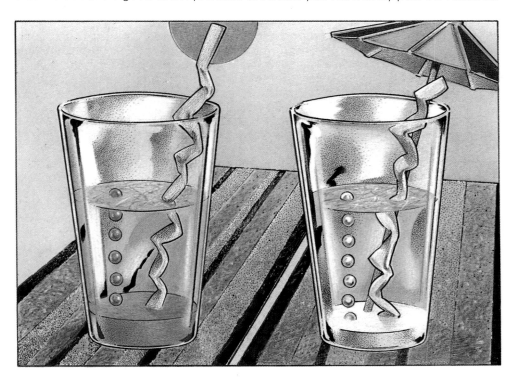

tan you already have. However, on burning, the skin almost immediately activates a few natural defences. Melanin, the skin's tanning ingredient, is present in small quantities in the skin's upper layers and a small amount is activated in the first few hours of exposure, darkening the skin and affording some protection. The rest of the suntan is only seen after the first two or three days of sunning yourself, as other melanin granules are activated and transferred to the skin cells which make their way to the surface. The skin consists of several layers, of which the bottom layer is the most recently formed, and the top layers the oldest which are continuously being shed. The skin's life-cycle lasts from 21-28 days, during which time the newly formed bottom layer cells rise to the surface and are then sloughed off. The full lifespan of a tan is therefore around three to four weeks, by which time the melanin in the lowest levels of the skin has risen to the top as the last of the tan.

A second immediate defence to UVA and B rays is an increase in the rate at which new skin cells are formed so that the new, thicker skin acts as a barricade and changes the wavelength of the rays, preventing them from doing some of their damage. However, it is this method of self-defence that causes the leathery look often seen in the skins of older people who have spent a great deal of their time outdoors.

THE SKIN'S DEFENCE MECHANISMS

The natural defences of the skin are not adequate against sunburn. If they were, dark and black-skinned people would suffer no side effects. But not only can black people get quite badly sunburnt, they are also not immune from the long-term damage inflicted by UVA rays. Black skin does age more slowly than white skin because of its better natural defences, which is why so many middle-aged black people have such enviably unlined skin, but exposure to the sun still speeds up ageing. At the same time, the incidence of skin cancer in black people is much lower than in white.

It is important to continue using suntanning lotions, even after you have acquired the desired tan. While the formation of melanin in the skin can protect against further burning, unless you take sunbathing to extreme lengths, it affords little or no protection against premature ageing. Albert Kligman, one of the world's top research dermatologists at the University of Pennsylvania, insists that once you are tanned, the level of the tan can be maintained with comparatively limited exposure to direct sun, and that the repeated use of protective sunscreening products provide the best guard against premature ageing of the skin. In short, once you are tanned, you could maintain the colour by using a **higher degree** of suntan protection than before, and this would have the added benefit of preventing your skin from ageing and wrinkling ahead of time. This advice contrasts strongly with the usual recommendations that you lower the protection level once you have browned.

WHAT IS A TAN?

A tan is the stimulation of the production of melanin following an attack by UV rays on the skin. Melanin, once activated, is distributed throughout the skin to act as a defence against further attack. The skin of black people is also coloured by melanin, although this is distributed evenly throughout the lifetime of the skin. In pale-skinned people melanin lies in the lower skin layers like a spoonful of honey at the bottom of a glass of milk; only when it is agitated does the milk turn honey-coloured.

Myth breaker
You will not tan deeper or faster if you have been burnt. Your skin will peel off and you will have to start again.

Myth breaker
IT IS NOT TRUE that tanned skin is immune to further damage by sun exposure. Melanin does protect against further burning, but gives no protection against premature ageing. ALWAYS use a lotion on tanned skin, and ideally one with a higher protection level.

Tip: don't be mean!
Never skimp on sun
products; a couple of tubes
will barely last for a
fortnight's holiday by the
sea.

Opposite: *The tender
spots on breasts,
collarbones and shoulders,
on lips, cheeks and nose,
on eyelids and scalp are
especially prone to sun
damage. Like plants behind
glass, they need a tough
barrier against the
elements; total sunblocks,
such as thick white zinc
oxide paste, give 100 per
cent protection.*

THE USE OF SUNTANNING PRODUCTS

Suntanning products slow down the effects of the sun's rays, giving the skin time to activate melanin without suffering the worst side effects — burning, blistering and peeling, the last of which results in your tan ending up in great chunks on your towel. They help you to acquire an acceptable colour without the brick-red highlights, and they also help to minimize any long-term damage. **It is important to remember that if your skin is absorbing enough sunlight to produce a tan, it is also absorbing enough energy to damage it.**

There are no products which can make you tan without sunlight. They are all skin dyes of one kind or another, usually either a chemical called dihydroxyacetone (DHA) or a natural staining ingredient such as extract of black walnut. DHA gives no protection from UV light at all, so do not be deceived into thinking your skin is protected by synthetic fake tans. Black walnut may be worth considering as it gives mild protection. Many people like to start their holiday with a fake tan, thereby avoiding the temptation to overdo it; they should still use sun protection throughout the day on top of the fake tan.

SUN PROTECTION FACTORS (SPFs)

All proprietary suntan products are labelled with Sun Protection Factors or SPFs, devised to inform you how much protection you can expect. Unfortunately, different companies arrived at their SPFs in slightly different ways, and one company's SPF2 is by no means identical to that of another. Even the methods used to test different levels of SPF are not standardized.

Sun protection factors themselves are ingredients suspended in lotions, oils or creams, usually about 5% of active ingredient to lotion, depending on the strength of protection. According to Dr F. Greiter, who devised the earliest sun protection factors, one problem with tanning is that more and more ingredients react with sunlight to cause allergies, known as photo-reactions or photo-allergic reactions. For this reason simple formulas are preferable to products with a vast range of different sunscreen ingredients.

As the SPFs vary so greatly, confusion remains as to the best choice of sun-tanning products. Guidelines which state that SPF2 means you can stay in the sun twice as long as without protection are helpful, although that rule of thumb seems to disintegrate slightly as you move up the scale. Some manufacturers misleadingly call their SPF 8 and 9 "sunblocks", while others define an SPF of 15 or 20 more accurately as having a high degree of protection. In addition, it is difficult to know how long you can stay in the sun to start with, before multiplying the time by 2 or 20.

Confusion about SPFs will remain until a standard method of assessment has been agreed upon. Most sunscreen evaluations are based on a method devised by Professor Rudolf Schulze in Germany in 1956. He calculated how long it would take a skin to burn *without* a sunscreen (say, 5 minutes) and how long it took to burn *with* a sunscreen (say, 20 minutes); by dividing 20 by 5, he arrived at an SPF of 4. However, everybody tans and burns differently, and the SPF figures arrived at by the manufacturers vary according to the number of people used in the tests.

Albert Kligman, an authority on tanning, maintains there need be only three categories of sun protection: Minimal (SPF 2 and 3), Moderate (SPF 4-6) and Maximum (above 6), adding that even very high SPFs filter out only 90% of the UV

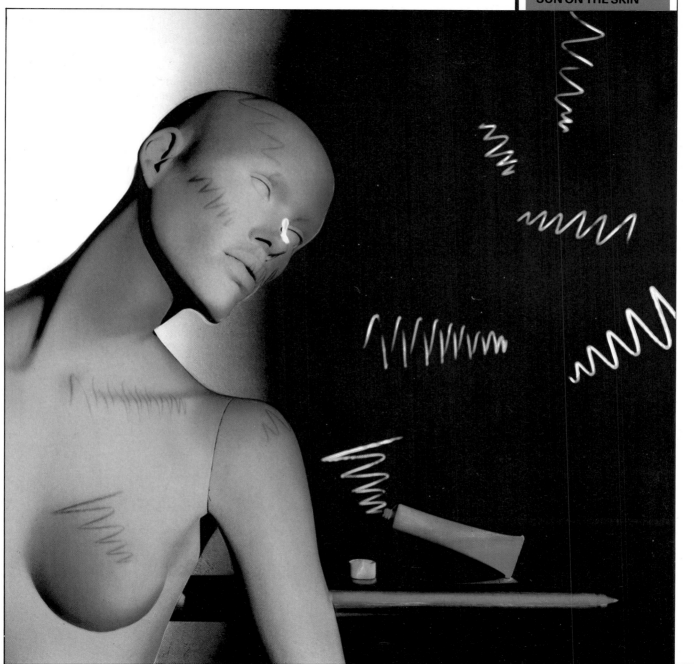

Warning: photo-sensitivity
Some skins respond strongly to sunlight, and allergic reactions can be triggered by the sun through glass; certain medications and foods can accelerate photo-sensitivity.

Fair skins are highly sensitive to sun; the pale-freckled Irish/Scottish and the fair English complexions, especially, peel within a few minutes of strong sun. Both need maximum sunscreens. The Scandinavian blonde tans more easily with less peeling, and though she may get away with moderate sun protection, she is better advised to use maximum.

rays. The Food and Drugs Administration in the United States have made similar recommendations, although they have added a fourth category, "Ultra". As Kligman said, "Only the Americans could come up with something higher than maximum!"

SKIN SENSITIVITY

Skin can be divided into six different categories as far as sun sensitivity and tanning ability are concerned (see chart overleaf). The typical Irish or Scottish complexion is the very fair skin which burns easily, often with severe and painful after effects, and followed by extensive peeling. This type of skin, very pale in colour and usually associated with blue eyes and freckles, hardly ever achieves a satisfactory tan; it is also the most **vulnerable to skin cancer.** Large numbers of the Scottish and Irish immigrants who settled in Australia during the last century passed their fair and sensitive skin on to their descendants; today it is quite common to see people with the facial scars left after the removal of skin cancer.

The so-called English skin type also burns easily and severely and has difficulty in tanning, with an accompanying tendency to peel. Characteristically, this skin type is fair, with red or blonde hair, and blue, hazel or even brown eyes; it is as prone to skin cancer as the very fair Irish skin type.

Average fair skin is not necessarily synonymous with tanning difficulties and easy burning; the typical Scandinavian blonde usually tans quite happily, with only minor burns, if lotions of moderate protection levels are faithfully applied.

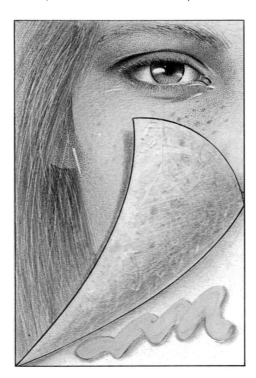

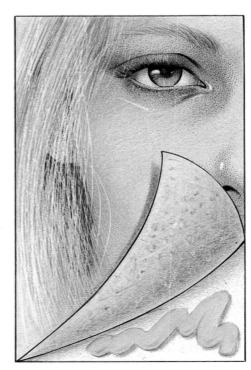

People with light brown skin, dark brown hair and dark eyes – the Mediterranean and Hispanic types – are the lucky ones. They tan easily, with moderate protection, showing immediate signs of darkening skin after a couple of hours of sun exposure, depending on the skin's natural brown pigmentation. Burns are minimal, and a strong tan will be apparent after a week. Brown-skinned people from the Middle East and the Indian subcontinent, as well as American Indians, tan more easily still, reacting to a few hours of sun with a distinct tan. The black skin of Africans and West Indians does darken and change colour after some hours in the sun, especially on people who are not used to strong sun; in these cases, burns can occur, but the dangers are infinitely less than with fair skins.

SUNBLOCKS

A total sunblock is often no such thing. Check the package to see if it guarantees total protection against UV rays, for only then is it a sunblock. You should consult your doctor on sun products if you have sensitive skin or a skin condition where sunlight could be dangerous. Zinc oxide, available from chemists, is a complete sunblock, but as it is a thick white paste it hardly looks flattering. Commercial sunblocks all contain either zinc oxide or titanium dioxide.

How much sun *you* can tolerate depends on the amount of melanin your skin can produce. A tan is determined genetically, and you can do nothing to alter the genes. You *can* bring out the positive aspects of a pale translucent skin.

Fact: Vitamin D
Osteomalacia, or bone fragility, especially in older people, is due to lack of vitamin D without which calcium cannot be absorbed. The vitamin is manufactured by the action of sunlight on the skin and is also present in foods such as milk and cheese, herrings and kippers.

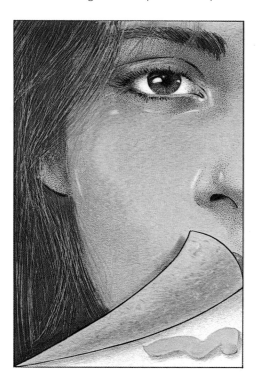
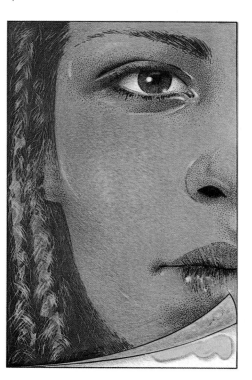

Dark-coloured
Mediterranean and Middle Eastern skins peel only slightly at average sun exposure. Moderate protection levels are generally advisable, though minimum sun-screens are acceptable on very dark types. Black skins, like West Indians and Africans, are the ONLY ones to tolerate minimum sun protection.

SUN SENSITIVITY AND TANNING

SKIN TYPE	TAN CAPACITY	BURNS	PEELS	EXPOSURE TIME Minus protection/Sunscreen		COMMENTS
Irish/Scottish: very fair skin, freckles, blue eyes	Very difficult	Easily	Almost always	10 min	MAXIMUM SPF: 20 min	Skin goes red; forget about tanning
English: fair skin, red/blonde hair, blue, hazel or brown eyes	Difficult	Easily	Usually	10 min	MAXIMUM SPF: 40-60 min	Will tan if protected; can tolerate an extra 10 min daily
Scandinavian: white skin, blonde hair, blue, green or brown eyes	Good	Moderately	Rarely	15 min	MODERATE SPF: 1 hour +	Depending on natural colours, skins can tolerate increasing exposure; strong tan visible after 1 week
Mediterranean/Hispanic: white or light brown skin, dark hair and eyes	Easy	Minimally	Rarely	15 min	MODERATE SPF: 2 hours +	
Middle Eastern/ American Indian: brown skin, hair and eyes	Easy, strong	Rarely	Rarely	20-25 min	MINIMUM SPF: 2 hours +	Reacts within a few hours of exposure, darkening distinctly
West Indian/African: black skin, eyes and hair	—	Rarely	Rarely	20-25 min	MINIMUM SPF: 2 hours +	Remember protection; burns can be painful and damaging

Fact: black myth
According to classical mythology, the black population was created by Phaeton, son of Apollo. He drove his father's sun chariot one day and lost control of the fiery horses; the chariot hurtled through the sky, setting the earth on fire and blackening the skins of the Ethiopians!

BLACK SKIN AND THE SUN

Black skin is extremely well equipped to deal with the sun. The colour pigment is melanin, as in white skin, but it is produced in larger particles and is always evenly distributed around the skin, and therefore constantly able to defend it from UV light. The outer layer of black skin is thicker, and the rate at which skin cells are produced is faster, both mechanisms which are inactive in white skins until exposed to UV light. The colour pigment in black skin can absorb much more UV radiation and can deal better with the "free radicals", which damage the DNA, elastin and collagen of white skin. Black skin ages much more slowly, hence the unlined faces of many middle-aged black women, and black skins are much less prone to skin cancer than white.

Black skin also has a better vaso-dilatory system, dealing much more efficiently with heat. There are 550 sweat glands per centimetre in the average white American skin, 600 in black American, 700 in black African and West Indian, and 740 sweat glands in every square centimetre of Hindu skin. This makes an appreciable difference in hot sun because a thick film of perspiration (about 1mm) provides some protection against the rays. Black skin also has more sebaceous glands, which secrete our skins' natural oiliness, and a mixture of sweat and sebum filters the ultraviolet light.

Black skin is better protected against the sun than white skin, partly because it is thicker, partly because it produces more melanin at a faster rate, and partly because it cools more readily, its natural mixture of sweat and oil giving some measure of natural sunscreening. In spite of all these plus factors, sunburn is not impossible, and can be a potential risk; black-skinned people who normally live an indoor life in towns and cities might easily get a painful shock after the first day on a tropical beach. The ageing process, although slower than on white skin, will also accelerate at repeated exposure to sun and after years of sunbathing. Even so, black skins are really the ONLY ones which can get away with always using the minimum level of sun protection in the Tropics, and none at all in Northern climates.

SUN IN HOT CLIMATES

Generally, higher levels of sun protection are necessary the nearer you go to the Equator where the sun's rays are hitting the Earth at right angles and are therefore less filtered by the atmosphere. Temperature and latitude are good guides for planning your tanning programme. If you have an Irish/Scottish or English skin type, you might just get away with moderate levels of protection during an average summer at Scarborough or Brighton, though maximum levels offer better protection. For a holiday in the Bahamas or Morocco, you MUST include plenty of complete sunblocks and products with maximum protection levels.

THE BEST POSSIBLE COLOUR

Be realistic about your skin tone. If you are born with pale, freckly skin and reddish hair, the only really good tan you are likely to acquire will come out of a bottle. Even if you do tan reasonably well, it may be advisable to combine certain elements of fake and real tan to get the best possible effect with the minimum of damage. Why not make a feature out of being pale?

FAKE TANS

These will probably contain either DHA or natural extracts, both of which are completely safe, but variable in colour and realism according to the base. The most effective and realistic DHA products are those incorporated in the so-called oil-in-water system. Before applying a DHA product, make sure that your skin is scrupulously clean, as this helps towards an even colour, and that the product has not deteriorated. Stored in a cool place, DHA products will keep their qualities for a *maximum* of two years. One interesting side effect of DHA is an improvement in acne as reported by many acne sufferers.

It is important to differentiate between a product which is a one-off pre-holiday application and one with a gentle tinting effect which will also protect the skin from UV rays. Products with natural extracts achieve a gradual effect over a period of two weeks. The Body Shop Cocoa-Butter Suntan Lotion is based on an extract of black walnut which slowly colours the skin brown, while the cocoa butter moisturises and conditions the skin and also gives mild protection against burns. Used daily for about ten days before your holiday it will gently tint the skin and prepare it for the onslaught of sun, sea and wind that will otherwise cause dryness and peeling.

Studies on extract of walnut reveal some advantages over DHA as a fake tanning agent. Both react with the protein in the top layers of the skin to form a coloured

Danger: don't do it!
Never sunbathe at midday; the sun is at its fiercest and your dermal tolerance at its lowest; sunbathe in the morning and in late afternoon, if you must acquire a tan.

Warning: brown is unhealthy
An article in *Vogue* in 1903 described a "nut brown" maid as being the picture of health, but warned that a tan and sunburn were uncomfortable and a detriment to appearance.

compound, but unlike DHA, walnut extract would appear to stimulate some defences against UV rays. Walnut extract products can generally be expected to have a moderate protective level as well as a fake tan element and can be used on normal skins both before and during the holiday.

DHA fake tan products do not normally contain sunfilter agents, so always check the instructions. They do not protect you from burning, and repeated applications of some brands could leave you a strange colour. A fake tan, whether based on DHA or walnut extract, will last as long as the outer layers of the skin – about a week at most. When the dead skin cells are shed, so is the fake tan. DHA products also wear off more quickly if you indulge in very hot baths and saunas on a regular basis.

SUNBEDS

The second most obvious way of arriving on holiday with a credible colour and speeding up the outdoor tanning process is to use a sunbed. Any claim by salon operators and beauticians that sunbeds "filter out harmful rays" should be viewed with suspicion. Any rays strong enough to encourage a tan must by definition have enough energy to damage the skin. Beware any establishment that allows you to use the equipment without guidance and supervision.

Most sunbeds use UVA light, and the main side effect from regular use may be premature ageing of the skin. Research into the long-term effect is incomplete and in spite of disapproval by dermatologists, there is no evidence that conclusively links skin damage with the regular use of sunbeds.

UVA tanning does not cause the skin to thicken like natural sunbathing, and your light sunbed tan will not protect you against burning during the first few days on the beach. Before using a sunbed, study a few guidelines, although these should be clearly explained to you by the sunbed operator:

1. Protect your eyes with goggles, or keep them shut.
2. Make sure there is an automatic switch or timer – and that it works – either to wake you up if you fall asleep, or to switch off the bed at the end of the session. Sunbed burns are very unpleasant.
3. Timing is approximately the same as for natural sunlight: 10 minutes for very delicate skin, 15 for average, 20-25 for very strong or dark skin.
4. If you are taking tetracycline antibiotics, water tablets or certain tranquillisers, a sunbed may produce a rash. Women on the contraceptive pill or those who are pregnant run the risk of developing chloasma (harmless blotches) around the face.
5. Thoroughly wash off all perfume and cosmetics. Do not apply suntan lotions; the ingredients could react with the UV rays to cause burning or allergic reactions.
6. Skin that is already slightly tanned or has been tanned before has a higher tolerance. If you usually sunbathe in a bikini and decide to use a sunbed without any clothes on, gauge the exposure time according to the paler areas.
7. Remember to use sunscreen products with adequate protection levels before you go on to the beach or into natural sunlight.

THE NATURAL TAN

Always buy your suntanning products before you set off on holiday, and always buy a generous supply. Although most commercial products are widely available at popular resorts, they can be prohibitively expensive, and in any case there is little point in

Warning
Psoriasis and eczema:
These conditions often improve on exposure to sun, but sometimes the opposite occurs. Obtain medical advice on the proper sunscreen preparation before sunbathing.

Warning: banish perfumes
Perfumes – and hand and body lotions containing scent – can react badly on exposure to sun, causing allergies or brown skin patches. Reserve perfume for evening wear, and moisturise the skin during the day with cocoa butter lotions.

trying to repair the damage after it has been done or in staggering around with red, peeling skin at best, agonizing burns at worst, in any case ruining several days of the holiday. Provided that you start off with the proper sun protection, you will probably avoid burns and painful blisters altogether, as well as saving yourself money.

In spite of well-founded warnings against the dangers of suntanning, most people feel that the psychological benefits of returning from holiday with a tan far outweigh any long-term side effects. This is probably true for the one annual holiday of two or three weeks, but people who indulge in round-the-year or all-summer outdoor sports should remember that, even if they are not actually sunbathing, they are still exposed to continual UV rays.

The array of sunscreen products available from chemists and beauty shops is unnecessarily bewildering and can be condensed into three broad categories. If you have very fair or very sensitive skin (Irish/Scottish or English complexion), you should buy two kinds of sun protection: Maximum (above SPF 6) and Moderate (SPF 4-6). Our PABA Sunscreen Lotion is a Moderate protective lotion, containing PABA sunscreens, vitamin E and glycerine, a moisturising ingredient which prevents drying out of the skin. You will probably achieve the best — and safest — colour by acclimatizing yourself to strong sun with a maximum sunscreen and a broad-brimmed hat for the first few days; you may then be able to drop to moderate protection level, but if your skin is very sensitive, you will be well advised to wear a hat thoughout the holiday.

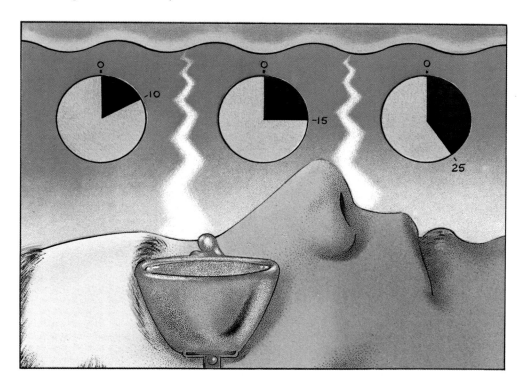

Fact
Salaman's Sensometer: This is a scientific test which measures our reaction to sun at different ages. We are most resistant at 3½-5 years, 13-17 years and 50-60 years; and most vulnerable at 6-8 years, 25-30 years for women, 30-35 for men.

Sunbeds *can lay the foundations for a holiday tan and help to maintain it afterwards. The ultraviolet rays will not burn provided you regard the tanning session exactly as if you were lying on the beach: no more than 10 minutes for very fair and white skins, 15 minutes for olive and light brown skins, and up to 25 minutes for dark brown and black skins. NEVER use tanning lotions and ALWAYS wear goggles.*

Skins which tan fairly easily (Scandinavian and Mediterranean/Hispanic) should be protected with a Moderate sunscreen product from the beginning; depending on skin sensitivity, the lotion can be continued throughout or replaced later with a Minimum level sunscreen. Black skins are the only ones that can risk using minimal protection all the time; it is unwise to do entirely without, and a sunscreen of Moderate level rather than Minimum will offer a greater degree of protection, against burning in the short term and against premature ageing in the long term.

SUN ON THE FACE

The face is the most important part of the body as regards sun protection. It is exposed to the elements all the year round, and facial skin is the first to show the lines and wrinkles of premature ageing. It begins to age in the early twenties while the skin on the buttocks, which are rarely exposed, is smooth and supple well into middle age. You may feel that the best protection you can give your face is to keep it out of the sun at all times and use fake tans for colour.

Perhaps the best overall advice is to use a high level of sun protection – protect your face from the sun with a hat, thick white cream or Body Shop products, according to the fairness of your skin. Your face usually tans more quickly than your body because it has been exposed to sunlight much more often.

Any part of the body with little fat is more vulnerable to burning and wear, hence the tendency of noses to turn a bright agonizing red and peel – often quite literally at the drop of a hat. Re-apply sun protection frequently on your face, especially on the nose, and in sunny tropical areas you may need a total sunblock, such as zinc oxide, to protect your nose in the middle of the day.

The delicate skin around the eyes is particularly vulnerable to ageing, and squinting into the sun can appear to deepen wrinkles because the sun outlines them as accurately as a red pen. The eyes themselves can suffer from prolonged exposure on a beach, boat or snowy mountain – after a day at sea staring across the bright water many sailors experience a "tunnel vision" effect. Apart from the possibility of eye strain, very bright sunlight is uncomfortable, so remember sun glasses. They protect the skin round the eyes better than creams, which in any case should not be taken too close to the eyes.

Lips are another particularly sensitive area. Many people suffer an allergic reaction to the sun which causes herpes (weeping cold sores) around the lips. The only prevention for this is a total sunblock, and if you are a herpes sufferer you should never venture into the sun without a zinc oxide cream or a total sunblock lipsalve. Natural remedies for this condition include finely grated raw apple, fresh lemon juice or a double-strength infusion of sage and plain yoghourt; the latter is also recommended for dry, cracked cold sores. Dry and cracked lips after a day spent in the open can be treated with an ordinary lipsalve. The Body Shop Lip Balm is a creamy gel-like emulsion with apricot, coconut, banana or cherry oils. Lavender aromatherapy oil has been successful in the treatment of cold sores.

A sunburnt scalp can be painful, and it is an easy part of the body to forget. While your face and body are protected with lotions or clothes, the scalp may be fully exposed all day. Hats, parasols or beach umbrellas are the only answers.

YEAR-ROUND SUN PROTECTION

As the evidence on sun damage to the skin builds up, a body of thought proposes sunscreens for year-round use. The proposition that sunscreens should be included in moisturisers, foundations, lipsticks and hair products might be greeted with a hollow laugh in Britain where we probably do not see enough sun to do ourselves any damage. That is why English women's complexions are famous. In our dull, damp climate there is relatively little sun to damage and dry out the skin. However, in the United States an increasing number of companies are beginning to incorporate some form of sun protection into everyday products.

Sun care should be an everyday routine in many other countries. In the Mediterranean and the East women often look older than their age, even those with skins dark enough to have some natural protection against UV light. In time, sunscreens can be expected to become standard in cosmetic products, and Body Shop anticipates a range of colour cosmetics with UV filters.

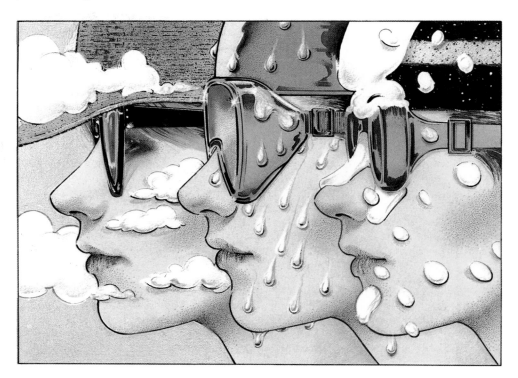

Warning: don't do it! Deodorant soaps can react with sun to produce a rash on the skin.

Sun rays *can cause burns even when you don't feel hot. More than 30 per cent of the ultraviolet rays can penetrate cloud cover, and though water cools the skin, it also acts as a magnifying glass, sometimes causing burns severe enough to blister and become infected. On snow-covered mountains, the sun burns particularly fiercely with 85 per cent of the rays being reflected from the snow.*

Fact: did you know?
About 50% of the sun's damaging UVB rays can penetrate terry cloth.

More and more people spend time outdoors, on holidays and business, in hotter, drier climates. They are getting more sun over the year than before, and for them it is probably worth thinking about all-year sun protection.

APPROPRIATE PROTECTION

The inclusion of a sunscreen in an everyday product like a moisturiser is often at such a low level that it is hardly effective. While sun products in the form of cream or lotion are applied repeatedly during the day in order to maintain their efficacy, few people re-apply their moisturiser. If you spend a great deal of time outside in a hot country, the normal rules of suntanning and sun protection products apply. Dermatologists agree that even in the Northern hemisphere low levels of sun protection in everyday products are highly commendable.

A moisturiser with a natural sun filtering element like Aloe vera is undoubtedly a good choice. As the trend towards the inclusion of a sunscreen in everyday cosmetic products gathers momentum, Aloe vera could become an ever more important ingredient because of its natural moisturising and emulsifying properties. One of the reasons for the slow emergence of sunscreens in cosmetics is due to the difficulty experienced in research laboratories of combining a sunscreen with other in-gredients, especially if these are perfumed; they occasionally fail to emulsify or they discolour within a short time.

It would appear that carrot may contain a natural element of sunscreen; Carrot Facial Oil and, therefore, Carrot Moisturising Cream would be appropriate products in this context. Apart from the sun-filtering possibilities of carrot, vitamin A in carotene is essential for healing and maintaining skin growth; it is used as an aftersun treatment for rough skin.

It is too early to evaluate year-round sun protection in cooler climates, but the evidence so far is favourable. Dermatologists agree that ingredients which filter UV light are more important in the fight against wrinkles than any of the various "miracle" ingredients that periodically go in and out of fashion.

STAYING IN THE SHADE

Staying in the shade is not as simple as it might appear. UV rays bounce back at you off water, sand, white surfaces and walls, and off snow. Studies in the United States have shown that fresh snow reflects 85% of the sun's rays, while dry sand reflects 17% and dry grass 2.5%. Some of the sun's rays can be conducted through materials. The same studies estimated that 50% of the UV light penetrate an average beach umbrella, 30-50% get through cloud and 20-40% get through a wet T-shirt, especially in the middle of the day.

It is unwise to rely too much on a beach umbrella for protection. As the sun moves overhead so does the patch of shade from your parasol, and it is easy to fall asleep in the shade only to wake up and find yourself grilled like a well-done steak.

Tight, slightly translucent synthetic clothing, which includes some swimsuits, allows penetration of some UV light. Loose cotton is the ideal clothing under a strong sun, as it lets through no UV light. The Arab burnoose and djellaba are prime examples of clothing adopted for maximum protection, and both men and women in the Middle East keep their bodies and heads well covered in cotton clothing.

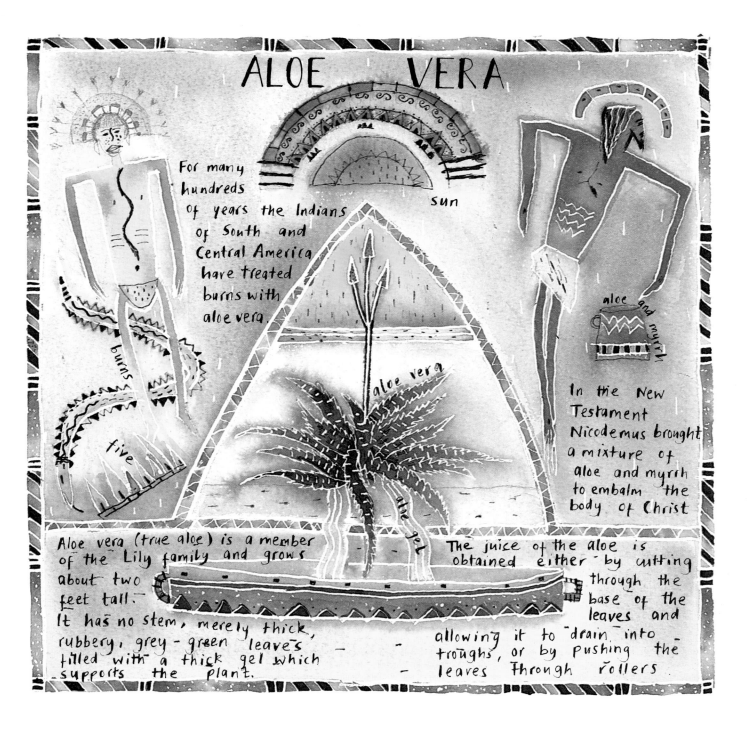

ALOE VERA

For many hundreds of years the Indians of South and Central America have treated burns with aloe vera.

sun

burns

fire

aloe vera

aloe gel

aloe and myrrh

In the New Testament Nicodemus brought a mixture of aloe and myrrh to embalm the body of Christ

Aloe vera (true aloe) is a member of the Lily family and grows about two feet tall. It has no stem, merely thick, rubbery, grey-green leaves filled with a thick gel which supports the plant.

The juice of the aloe is obtained either by cutting through the base of the leaves and allowing it to drain into troughs, or by pushing the leaves through rollers

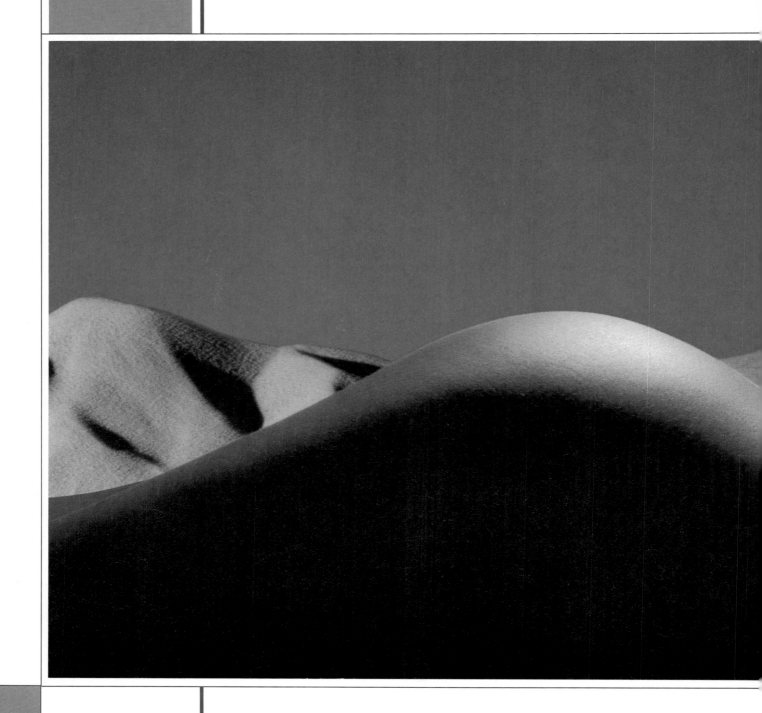

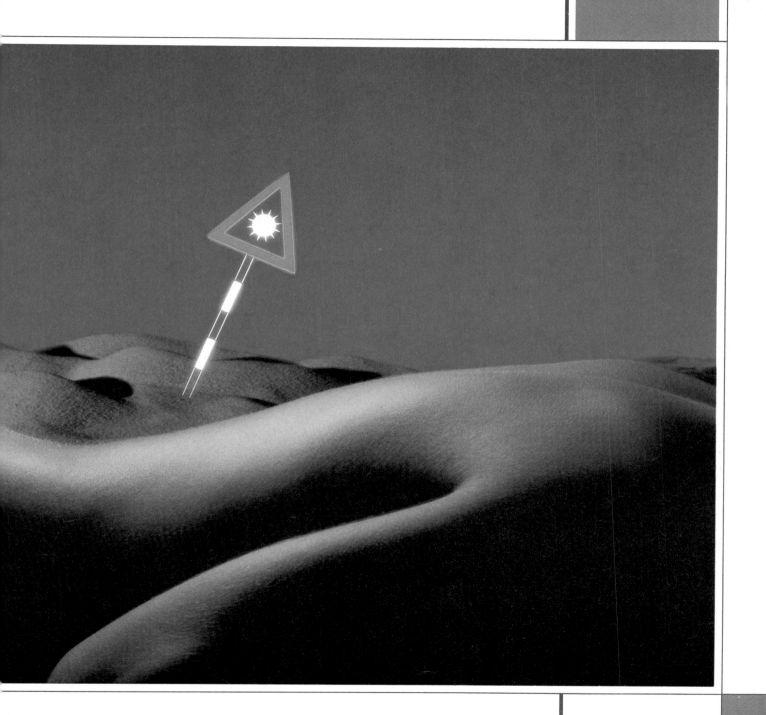

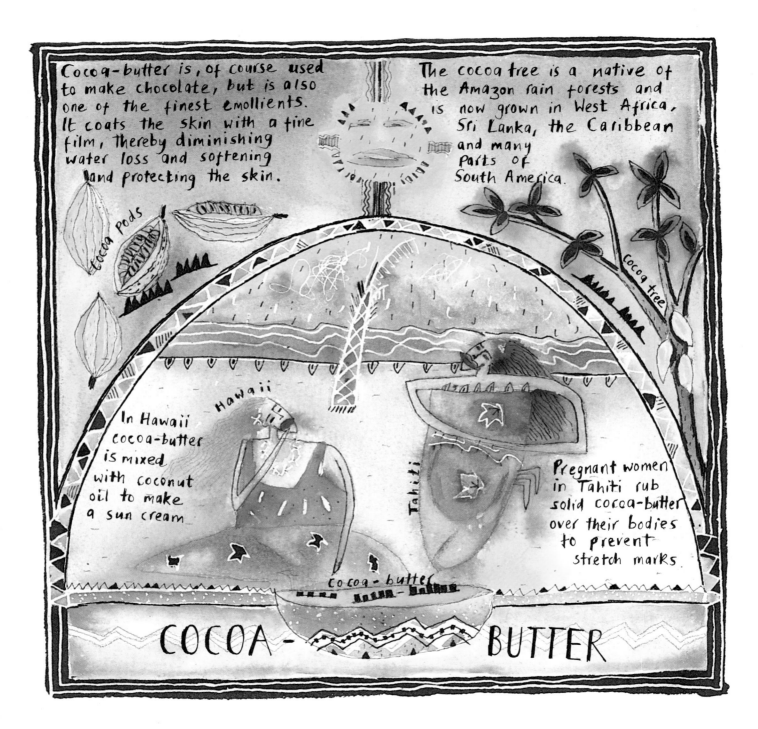

Cocoa-butter is, of course used to make chocolate, but is also one of the finest emollients. It coats the skin with a fine film, thereby diminishing water loss and softening and protecting the skin.

The cocoa tree is a native of the Amazon rain forests and is now grown in West Africa, Sri Lanka, the Caribbean and many parts of South America.

Cocoa Pods

Cocoa tree

In Hawaii cocoa-butter is mixed with coconut oil to make a sun cream

Hawaii

Tahiti

Pregnant women in Tahiti rub solid cocoa-butter over their bodies to prevent stretch marks

cocoa - butter

COCOA - BUTTER

SUNNIES

The skin over the eyelid is the thinnest, and even with the eyes shut you risk eye strain in bright sunlight. The skin round the eyes is also most prone to wrinkles. Special goggles, known as "Sunnies" and "Super Sunnies", protect and fit over the eyes without leaving white areas.

SUN GLASSES

Buying sun glasses is as confusing as buying suntan lotions. Technical terms on labels, such as photochromatic, polarizing, gradient, scratch-resistant, shatter-proof and so on leave you wondering exactly what you are paying for, and what exactly you need. Fashion also plays an important part in sun-glass design, with manufacturers and advertising campaigns tempting consumers to regard sun glasses as much as a fashion accessory as an optical necessity.

Polarizing lenses are the only ones which cut down reflected glare and the consequent eye strain encountered by anyone indulging in water sports, sailing and fishing. The Association of Dispensing Opticians recommends polarizing sun glasses for people spending a lot of time near or on water during the summer; remember that the lenses are only polarized if the labels clearly say so; not all Polaroid sun glasses, for example, have specific polarizing lenses.

Photochromatic lenses change colour and deepen as the light turns brighter. They are often more convenient than polarizing or ordinary sun glasses because the light hitting the eyes is more regulated, but the debate about their usefulness for driving continues. Because photochromatic lenses react to the UV rays in sunlight, which is already diminished inside a car, the sudden change in light intensity on emerging at speed from a darkish tunnel, for example, can present a hazard for the driver, and for other road users, as it may cause momentary blindness. However, for exactly the same reasons, photochromatic lenses are perfect for sunbathing and for general outdoor activities in summer as they protect the delicate skin round the eyes from UV light. For people with bad eyesight, it is also much more comfortable to use prescribed spectacles with photochromatic lenses instead of the clumsy sun visors attached with clips to an ordinary pair of spectacles.

Photochromatic lenses are often confused with the cheaper gradient lenses. These are simply glasses designed with darker glass or plastic at the top to block the sun, and lighter at the base for better visibility. They are generally adequate for normal wear. Fashion sun glasses may have any of these characteristics, but mainly they are intended as no more than an amusing fashion accessory while keeping your eyes shaded. They have no specific optical advantages. Every summer sees new designs, and major chemists and department stores offer a wide choice in styles ranging in price from the cheap to the wildly extravagant and from the "winged" style popular in the 1950's to speckled, checked or striped frames or solid colours of white, pink, yellow and blue; the lenses may be tinted rose, violet or blue-grey, and some are even spotted with contrasting colours.

One fairly recent development in sporting sun glasses uses a material called Crylon, which is claimed to be unbreakable and shatter-proof. They have tough, pliable frames and lenses; as they will not break or splinter during a fall, they are particularly suitable for ski-ing. However, they have no specific optical advantages, and the lenses tend to scratch easily.

Warning
Your sun glasses do not give proper protection if you can see your eyes when you look into the mirror.

Sunbathing can damage your health. *Forget about deep tans (see previous pages); they can be the forerunners of skin cancer and are always accompanied by dry skin, uneven colour patches and premature wrinkles.*

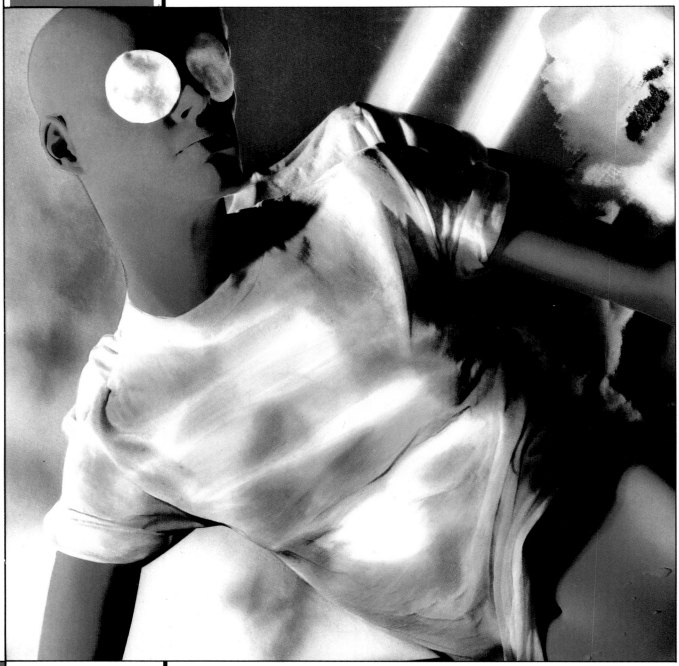

Anyone with sensitive eyes should consult an optician over the choice of sun glasses. Sensitivity to light usually also means sensitivity to one or more colours of the spectrum and you might pick the wrong colour lenses without professional advice. If you wear contact lenses, buy sun glasses from the optician.

SKI-ING

It is easy to forget about protection on a ski-ing holiday when you are wrapped up to the ears in thick clothing. The sun's rays are particularly fierce, partly because the UV rays are less filtered by the thin atmosphere in high mountains, and partly because reflected light from the snow combines with overhead light to assault the skin. A tanned face in the middle of February when everyone else looks white used to be considered a great morale booster, but is now passé. The long-term effects on your skin can be damaging. Always wear sun glasses or goggles, and always use a fairly high level of sun protection – moderate or maximum – depending on your skin type. If you suffer from sun-reactive lip sores, these will be particularly evident on ski-ing holidays so take a total sunblock lipsalve.

You will be sweating and falling over in the snow a great deal, and sun protection washes off very easily; re-apply the protection frequently or use a waterproof sunscreen. The wind and cold will also strip your skin of its essential oils and elasticity so be careful in the choice of a good moisturiser. Aloe Vera Moisturiser is particularly suitable, because its soothing and healing properties on chapped and burnt skin, including those exposed to X-rays, have long been known. Studies have shown that at the concentration of 1-2% of cream or lotion, Aloe vera also gives effective sunburn protection against burning UVB rays as it has a natural sunscreen ingredient, useful for less extreme conditions.

Fact: X-ray burns
Aloe vera has been used effectively in the treatment of X-ray burns, and at one time the US army stockpiled the cream for use against radiation burns after a possible nuclear attack.

SUN ON THE BODY

Different aspects relate to tanning the body than to tanning the face. Your body remains covered up far more than your face, and is therefore less likely to suffer long-term effects of sun damage. Going brown for a few weeks once a year on holiday *will* accelerate ageing of body skin, but minimally so.

For depth of colour before protection, you could use a lower level of sun protection on the body, or use a suntan oil rather than a cream or a lotion. In the United States, where the depth of a tan used to be a status symbol, most suntanning products are oils, which give less protection; in Europe, greater importance is laid on a healthy skin, and creams and lotions are preferred to oils.

Oils give less protection against UV light, being ineffective vehicles for sun-screens. They also have less substantiveness to the skin than creams and lotions which glide on smoothly, cover more thoroughly and are more easily absorbed. Very

Opposite: The sun is your enemy, *penetrating clouds to damage the eyes and burn fair skin even through a wet T-shirt. Its glare is reflected and magnified by snow, and even fluorescent lights in offices have been known to affect sensitive skins.*

Danger: frying in oil
If you rub yourself all over with olive or baby oil you will literally fry. This is because the glistening surface reacts like a magnifying glass to the sun's rays.

Tip: cool creams
Keep after-sun preparations – and other creams and lotions – cool and soothing by storing them in the fridge.

DIY tip: sun cream
A recipe for those who take home-made cosmetics seriously. *It has minimal sun protection value:*
100ml natural yoghourt
6 tablespoons water-dispersible lecithin
2 tablespoons sesame seed oil
2 tablespoons avocado oil
3 tablespoons water
1 tablespoon potato flour
Whisk all the ingredients in an electric blender until smooth.

often a lower level of protection in a cream or lotion will actually protect you better than an oil with slightly higher protection factors, but difficult to apply evenly.

Contrary to popular belief, **oils do not promote tanning.** Substances, known as photo-active ingredients, can be added to accelerate tanning. The best are probably those developed from bergamot oil, but in order to formulate a product with enough tanning accelerator to be effective, the ingredient must be added in sufficient quantities to cause photo-traumatic or photo-toxic reactions. Sensitive skin conditions, allergies and other side effects from the sun are even more likely to occur from a product with tanning accelerators. If you develop brown patches, a rash or any other unusual skin condition when using a product with a tan accelerator, you should change it immediately.

However, oils can be attractive as they add a glossy sheen to a tanned skin. Although they are not ideal tan protectors, products on the market have been formulated to overcome most of their disadvantages and can be pleasant over an established tan. The only oil with good inbuilt sunscreen properties is sesame seed oil, which can be used on its own on the beach. It is easily absorbed by the skin and has a pleasant, nutty scent.

HOME-MADE SUNTAN PREPARATIONS

You can have great fun making your own suntan preparations. Most of the ingredients are available from health food shops and good chemists; on holidays abroad keep an eye on local markets and bring back new ingredients to try.

Sun protection products belong to the 20th century and the Western world. In hot countries, the natives deliberately protect themselves from the sun and remain in the shade as much as possible. They also have stronger, darker skins better able to withstand the consequences of sun exposure. Middle Eastern women would be astonished if asked for a traditional recipe for suntan lotion: until fairly recently, they would not dream of appearing outside with anything more than a small patch of cheek visible.

The Tibetans, on the other hand, being vulnerable to the strong UV light in the Himalayas, did develop a suntan remedy which proved useful as a sunscreen. It was made from a mixture of tar and local tannin-rich herbs and was used effectively by mountaineers. However, as it tended to rust climbing equipment, its use has somewhat diminished!

Tea, made from a strong brew and left to infuse, is a recurrent theme in many home-made tanning products. Sesame seed oil is the usual sunfilter, as in this greasy, but very water-resistant oil for skins that tan easily: mix equal amounts of sesame seed and coconut oil (or almond oil) with 1 teaspoon of wheatgerm oil and a few drops of iodine. Coconut oil, white, semi-solid and lard-like, is an excellent emollient for cosmetic and suntan products, and for shampoos. It needs to be melted until liquid before being mixed with the sesame seed oil, but once blended will not harden. You can also substitute vitamin E for the wheatgerm oil and iodine.

For a super creamy, less greasy tanning cream, melt 25ml lanolin until liquid, then beat in 75ml sesame seed oil, 2 tablespoons of wheatgerm oil and 3 tablespoons of comfrey root water; beat thoroughly until the mixture has cooled.

For **sensitive skins**, warm 2 parts coconut oil with 1 part sesame seed oil until evenly blended; remove it from the heat, add a few drops of sandalwood oil and beat thoroughly. Store the oil in a bottle and shake it well before use.

Lotions for **skins which tan quickly** can be easily made by mixing 1 tablespoon of lemon juice into home-made mayonnaise or salad dressing consisting of 2 parts olive oil to 1 part vinegar, thoroughly shaken.

There is no scientific evidence to back up claims that oil and vinegar mixtures have any suntanning properties, but they do act as moisturisers of the skin and they are always readily at hand.

Other ingredients from the kitchen cupboard can be used for an exotic Tahitian tan; this recipe comes from the Tropics, and as it is invented for dark skins, it gives only minimal sun protection: put 25g of cocoa butter, 50ml of coconut oil and 25ml of sesame seed oil into a liquidiser and blend until evenly combined. Never use perfume in suntanning products, but a few drops of gardenia or pikake oil may be added for scent. The Australians use tea as a base in lotions for skins that tan reasonably well: leave 150ml of tea (made from 3 teaspoons of tea leaves) to infuse for 20 minutes, blend at low speed 50ml of lanolin, 50ml of sesame seed oil and a third of the tea until smooth; increase the speed and add the rest of the tea.

AREAS TO WATCH OUT FOR
Some parts of the body are more vulnerable than others to sun-damage. The bony bits suffer most — the lack of protective fat on shin and collarbones can mean quite agonizing burns and should be given special attention. Collarbones and shoulders are

The vulnerable areas are the ones you easily forget. The bony bits on the face, collar bones and shoulders — on the back as well as the front — and the nipples are the first to suffer under hot sun; cover them with frequent applications of sunscreen cream or lotion.

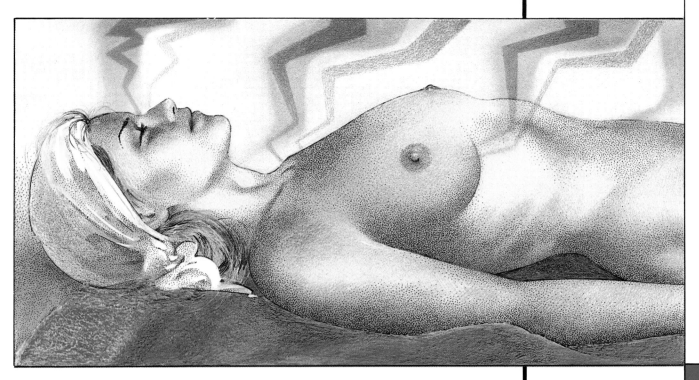

likely to burn on the first few days of your holiday, but they can be protected with zinc oxide. The most vulnerable areas are those which hardly ever see the sun, such as the nipples, breasts and bottoms, all of which can be protected with a higher SPF level, or by covering up with frequent applications of sunscreens or zinc oxide . If you develop a tan in one particular swimming costume or bikini, and then switch to a different costume, white areas will promptly burn and blister.

Burns on the soles of the feet will really cramp your style. Luckily, the thick skin there and on the palms of the hands take much longer to burn, and for most of the time you will probably be wearing some form of foot protection; however, if you are lying stretched out on your tummy sunbathing, you should remember lotion, on the soles as well as on the back of the knees.

Many people believe that lying on the beach or sunbathing in the garden is somehow ''worse'' for your skin than a suntan achieved through energetic outdoor activities. This mistaken idea is possibly a hangover from Victorian days and the strict moral views that lazing around was irresponsible and was bound to be punished. Whatever the reason, however, the conclusion is certainly wrong for your skin can burn just as easily when you are standing up or running around indulging in sports. It is particularly easy to get badly sunburnt from sailing and wind-surfing because while the sea breezes keep the skin cool, they do not in any way reduce the burning capacity of the sun's rays; often you do not realize how badly burnt you are until you are back on land.

The soles of the feet are tough but can still burn if unprotected. The bikini line, top of the thighs and the knees and back of the legs are more sensitive and liable to painful red patches and peeling.

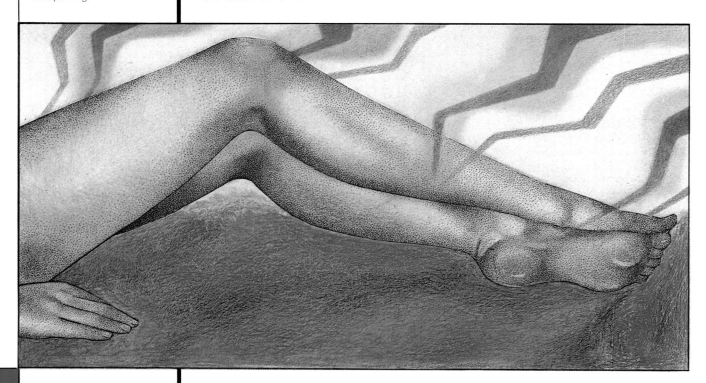

SUN ON THE HAIR

T he sun's effect on the hair is even more extreme than on the skin, mainly because the possibility of painful burning forces us to protect our bodies with clothes and lotions. As hair is composed of dead cells, we often forget about it.

The two main and obvious effects are drying and bleaching. Less is known about the chemical effect the sun has on hair and about the actual mechanism of that action. You should protect the hair by keeping your head in the shade as much as possible, by wrapping a towel round it on the beach or by wearing a hat. A few companies include sunscreens in their hair products, but very few, and their effectiveness is as yet unknown; future developments will probably mean sunfilters in many hair products to prevent dyed hair from changing colour and to minimize the drying effects of the sun.

Bleaching may sound attractive – phrases like ''sun-lightened'' or ''sunkissed'' hair spring to mind, but the effect can be quite disastrous on dyed and permed hair. People who have treated themselves to a lift with a head of highlights or a blonde rinse before holidays come back looking like peroxide blondes. Red hair dyes of all kinds, chemical and natural, fade very quickly in the sun, and dark hair may become peppered with grey. **If you regularly colour your hair you would be wise to leave it until after your holiday**.

A perm often has a bleaching and drying effect in itself, and exposing it to strong sunlight is a further harsh treatment. Plan to have a perm at least a month before your holiday. The drying effects of the sun can also make a perm less long-lasting, and your hairstyle, unless properly moisturised and protected, may lose shape and body earlier than it would otherwise have done.

MINIMIZING HOLIDAY HAIR-DAMAGE

Use a conditioner, which contains humectants to re-moisturise your hair and a mixture of polymers to protect the hair from heat, such as the Body Shop Hair Salad, which can be combed through the hair before sunbathing and rinsed off afterwards. It can also be used as a conditioning treatment in the evening.

After swimming, rinse all salt and pool chemicals out of the hair. There is no need to keep shampooing it, but rinse thoroughly with clear water. Blondes in particular may find that chlorine pool water gives the hair a greenish tinge.

SHAMPOOS AND CONDITIONERS

A frequency wash shampoo is appropriate for holidays in order to minimize stripping and drying effects. Conditioners should always be used. You should also consider a re-moisturising treatment to restore lost oils, body and shine. The main function of a conditioner is to make the hair more controllable, but for those extremes of dryness and brittleness associated with holiday hair, a more thorough re-moisturising

DIY tip: mosquito protection
A few drops of citronella added to a bottle of witch hazel can be used as an anti-mosquito splash; however, on sensitive skin it can cause an allergic reaction with the sun.

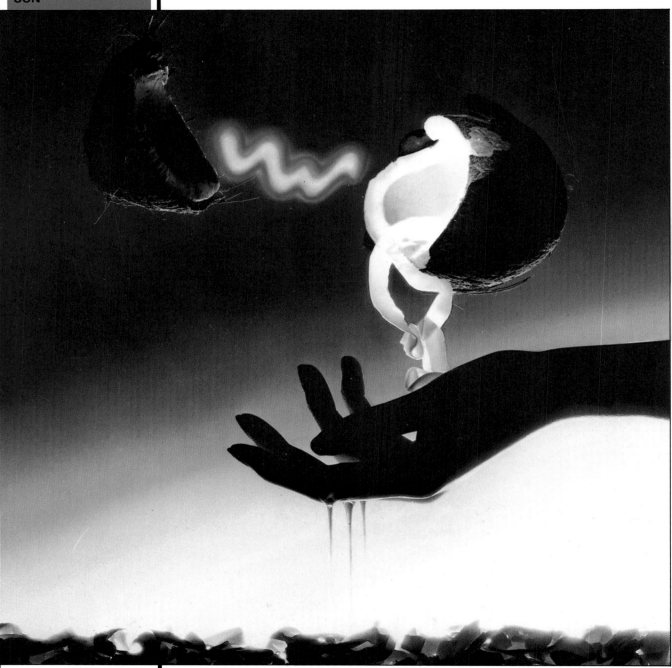

treatment is necessary. With time to spare, give your hair a truly special treatment with a hair pack or a product like Body Shop Henna Treatment Wax, which can be left on for half an hour.

TWENTY WAYS WITH HAIR GEL

Holidays give you ample opportunities to try out different hair styles and play around with your looks. Take hair gel with you – the Body Shop Hair Gel is based on coconut milk and a modern polymer – and experiment with some of these styles:

Afro Finger-dry with hair gel for a wet look and to combat frizziness.	**Plaits** Apply hair gel to each major strand for little-girl plaits to look smooth and sleek.
Blow Dry Massage hair gel into wet hair before blow drying to give volume and direction to any conventional hair style.	**Rock-a-billy** Keep quiffs and D.A's in place with hair gel.
Bob Hair gel spread lightly over the palms of the hands and smoothed over a straight hair style will have the same effect as a light hair spray.	**Scrunge** A "just-out-of-bed" look can be achieved with hair gel first smoothed, then tousled and scrunged while the hair is drying.
Braids Naturally curly hair, braided and beaded, remains sleek and smooth with an application of hair gel. Use it while braiding to speed up what is normally a time-consuming process.	**Set** Use hair gel as a combination of setting lotion and hair spray; apply to wet hair before setting on rollers for any classic set.
	Sleek For a smooth, wet look, rub hair gel into dry hair and comb flat with a fine-tooth comb while still damp.
Crimp An application of hair gel before crimping gives volume, protects the hair and cuts out hair sprays.	**Spike** Finger-dry and tweeze short hair into shape to get a "Johnny Fingers" look.
Crop Short hair can be tweezed into shape with hair-gelled fingers, tonged for a reed-like effect or brushed through for a casual appearance.	**Sunshade** Use hair gel to create a sun-shade from a fringe.
	Thirties Use hair gel on wet hair and comb it into the classic finger-wave vamp look.
Curly Maintain or twist permed or natural curls with a little hair gel applied to dry hair.	**Traditional** Use hair gel to hold partings in place on windy days.
Mohican Punk orange or pink crests remain erect with hair gel.	**Volume** Hair gel rubbed into the roots, then teased out gives volume to naturally dried hair.
Outrageous Styles that astound are common ground for only a pound (with apologies to William Blake).	**Windswept** Cover the ends of blow-dried hair with gel for a wet look, and brush it through for a windswept look.

Warning
Never use medicated sulphur as a hair dye. It can cause violent headaches and nose-bleeds.

Opposite: *Coconut oil is manna for a cracked and brittle skin which laps up the rich emollient drops to regain smoothness and elasticity.*

Fact: time consuming
A late 16th-century description details the extraordinary pains that fashionable Venetian ladies took to dye their dark hair. They would spend the night with the hair rubbed in a mixture of dried caul, egg yolks and honey, wash it in the morning in olive oil and retire for the day to the sun roof of the palazzo. Here they would don a solanna, a wide-brimmed straw hat without a crown, spread the hair over the brim and then, assisted by their maids, they would spend the whole day anointing it repeatedly with lotions containing saffron or medicated sulphur.

Opposite: Sunscorch can leave the skin as parched and brittle as a desert landscape. In shade, the skin's natural oils mixed with sweat create a moist protective surface film.

HERBAL HAIR COLOURS IN THE SUN

The sun has a role to play in hair colouring, most obvious in bleaching and blonding. Since the earliest days blonde hair has been sought after – and distrusted. Yellow was a fashionable hair colour among the Ancient Greeks and evoked the same criticism as peroxide blondes did until punk hair fashions extended the tolerance for obvious fakes. The Greek poet and comedy writer, Menander (342-291BC), is recorded as saying that women who bleached their hair were "outraging the character of gentlewomen, causing the overthrow of houses, the ruin of nuptials and accusations on the part of children". Clement of Alexandria took the equally pompous view that women who bleached their hair "became lazy in housekeeping, sitting like painted things to be looked at, not as if made for domestic economy". In ancient Rome, yellow hair was the mark of the prostitute, but when the Roman conquerors began to import blonde Scandinavian slave girls, the respectable society ladies felt forced to use saffron to dye their hair to compete for their husbands' affection.

Saffron has been prized since Solomon's times; it is obtained from the autumn crocus which grows wild in Asia Minor. Millions of flowers have to be collected by hand to provide one kilogram of saffron, and consequently it is extremely expensive. The essential oils contain a yellow dye which is water soluble and while unsuitable for the dying of fabrics, it is excellent as a natural hair colouring.

You can prepare your own saffron hair lightener by simply crushing the contents of a small pack of culinary saffron and adding 100ml of boiling water. Leave this to infuse, covered, for at least 5-6 hours in a warm place. Strain the infusion, add a squeeze of lemon juice and bottle the preparation. After shampooing and rinsing, pour about one third of the above quantity over the hair – for long and natural blonde hair, the saffron mixture can be diluted with an equal amount of water. The colour is immediate, but gradually washes out with shampooing. You can also use saffron hair lightener as a sun spritzer while you are sunbathing, to give interesting highlight effects to brown hair.

Sitting in the sun for long periods will do your hair no good, but if you use herbal dyes to bleach or blonde your hair, a few hours in the sun will heighten the effect.

AFTER SUN

After-sun care is as important as sun protection during the day. However careful you are on the beach, a day of sunbathing is the skin's equivalent to an army assault course, and follow-up care is necessary to restore the skin to peak condition.

Rinsing is the first step of after-sun care. It may not be necessary to use soap or a shower gel to remove dirt, but it is important to get rid of all salt deposits from sea water and chemicals from pool water as these, together with wind and sun, strip the

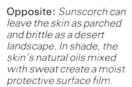

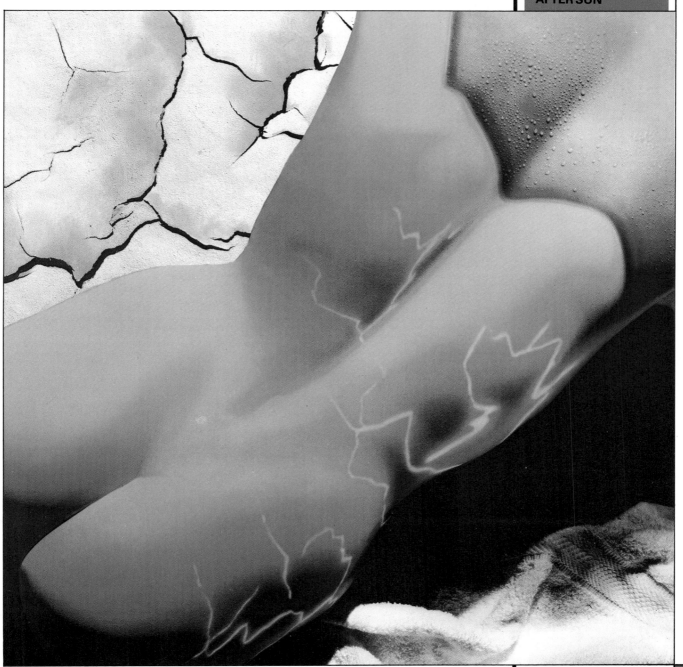

Fact, not fiction
Pool and tap water remove suntan preparations much more quickly than sea water.

Tip: moisturisers for men
Dry skin is as much a male as a female skin problem, even if male skin is tougher and takes longer to age. Moisturised after shaves are recommended as after-sun care for all male skins.

Dry facial skin *poses potential health dangers. Viewed on a horizontal plane, left to right, the top cell layer on thin-skinned, parched areas literally peels away in chunks. Dry skin reflects light poorly, making it dull and sallow; in extreme cases it cracks, especially round the mouth, leading to lip sores and other infections.*

skin of its vital moisture. After rinsing, apply a cooling and healing re-moisturiser to the face and to all parts of the body, smoothing on and massaging in a cream, oil or lotion to prevent the skin from drying out.

Dry skin (and all skin is made drier by sunbathing and swimming) is neither attractive nor healthy. The top layer of cells peel up at the edges and break away in chunks like worn rooftiles. Slightly dry skin feels "tight" and reflects light badly, which makes it look dull and lack-lustre, and very dry skin is prone to infection and irritations because the skin may crack enough to allow bacteria to invade the lower levels.

Although water is the ingredient missing from dry skin, long periods spent in the bath or pool will not help. Anyone who has spent a long time in water will be familiar with "waterlogged" skin, where it has sucked in water and developed a prune-like look. Most of this evaporates fairly quickly (leaving your skin drier than before), but in a waterfilled skin the cells expand, water creeps in between, and the normal barrier breaks down to make the skin vulnerable to infections.

The purpose of all moisturising creams, oils and lotions is to counteract dryness and keep the skin looking younger. Moisturiser is the greatest and probably the oldest beauty aid; it first saw the light of day as an all-purpose cold cream, made of olive oil and bees' wax to a recipe by the Greek physician Claudius Galen in AD 150. Science has been refining the recipe ever since. It was called cold cream because the water in the cream evaporated on contact with the skin, leaving a feeling of coolness.

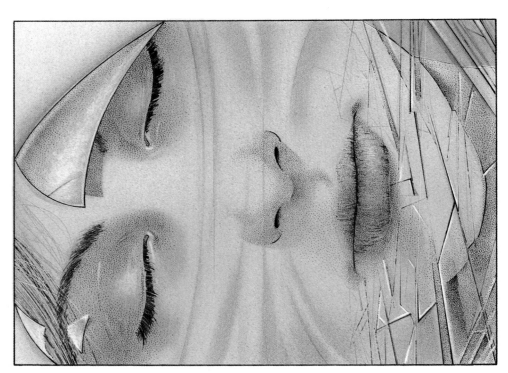

All externally applied oils and creams moisturise the skin by the inclusion of water in their formulations; the skin does not absorb the oil, but it creates a film over the surface, preventing the skin's own moisture from escaping, and softening the horny outer layers of the epidermis.

AFTER-SUN MOISTURISERS

The most effective moisturiser is probably lanolin. This is wool fat or grease; Australian sheep shearers roll in the lanolin left on the shearing table and come away with the skin as absolutely smooth and soft as a baby's. Lanolin makes excellent bases for ointments and creams due to its ability to absorb large amounts of water and liquids; it is closely related to human sebum. However, a significant minority react badly to lanolin, and must avoid any product containing this ingredient. Unless you are allergic to lanolin, the best treat for your face after a day in the sun is a super-rich moisturiser containing lanolin, like Rich Night Cream with Vitamin E, and Jojoba Oil Moisture Cream.

Other good moisturisers include cocoa butter, Aloe vera, honey and glycerine. Cocoa butter is a cream-coloured fatty wax which melts at body temperature; honey is one of the earliest known humectants, and glycerine is another excellent natural humectant, a by-product of soap-making. Glycerine is particularly good for healing chapped lips and hands.

A good after-sun preparation should also include a healing and soothing ingredient such as witch hazel. This extract is distilled from the bark of the hamamelis shrub and has long been known for its astringent and soothing properties. Products containing extract of witch hazel are suitable for skin irritated by insect bites and shaving, as well as sunburn. Chamomile is another good ingredient to use in after-sun preparations; the herb has long been used for medicinal purposes, especially to treat swellings and inflammations.

Straight oils do not work well as moisturisers unless they are combined in some way with water. This is why massage oils should always be rubbed in on slightly damp skin. Cooking oils are not really satisfactory, and while bath oils are less effective as moisturisers, they do help and can form part of your after-sun care. Body Shop Bath Oil is a combination of mineral oil and isopropyl myristate, a synthetic oil which is similar to certain parts of sebum and penetrates to dry skin. It is suitable as an after-sun conditioner, massaged on to damp skin after a bath.

B-carotene, otherwise known as provitamin A, and extracted from carrots, is increasingly used in after-sun care. Carotene is vital in promoting and maintaining healthy skin growth. When the skin is exposed to sun, the cells begin to speed up their natural reproduction processes in order to thicken the skin; carotene helps to calm this down, and thus to prolong the life of the tan. Carotene also has a mildly natural colouring effect which complements a tan, and recent research suggests that it might prove valuable in the treatment of UV-induced skin cancer. Body Shop products with carotene include Foaming Bath Oil, Carrot Facial Oil and Cream and Apricot Kernel Oil.

AROMATHERAPY

Aromatherapy can also be used as after-sun care and perhaps a holiday will give you the first opportunity to try this age-old health therapy. Its origins are lost in the mists

Fact: US approved
PABA formulated at 3% in cream formulations is still considered by the American army as the most effective sunscreen.

Tip: soothing lotions
After-sun preparations should contain moisturiser *and* soothing ingredients. The Body Shop Cocoa-Butter Hand and Body Lotion has as extra ingredients chamomile oil and extract of marigold to soothe and balm irritated skins. Rub it all over after a bath, while the skin is still damp.

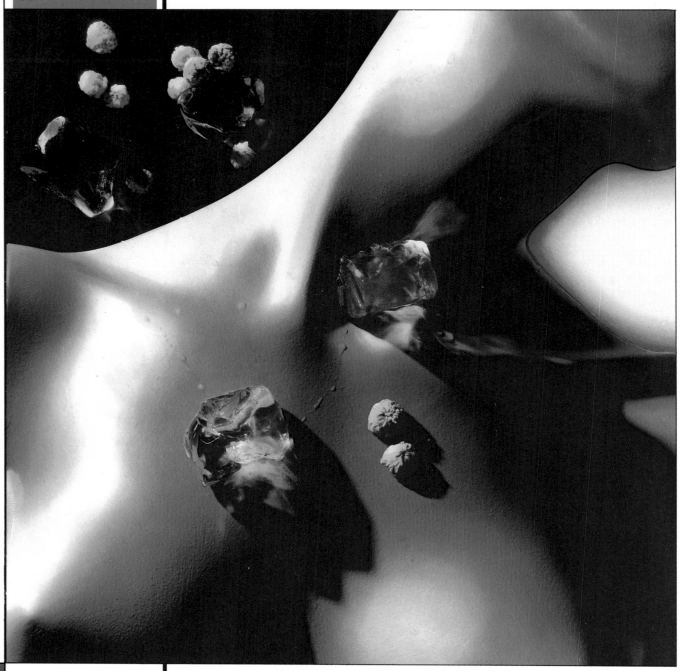

of time, though the ancient Egyptians certainly used it and relied on it as a restorer of the skin's natural oils and hormones, and as a soothing revitalizer of flagging muscles and strained nerves. Aromatherapy has become popular again with the renewed interest in alternative medicines; many salons employ aromatherapists trained in the different uses and benefits of the different essential oils.

For do-it-yourself aromatherapy, the oils can be inhaled or applied topically. For direct application, smooth the chosen oil sparingly over the area to be treated and massage it in gently. A particular oil may sting on application; if this happens, wash it off immediately with lukewarm water and change to another essential oil.

Chamomile oil is particularly beneficial for treating sunburns as it reduces redness and swelling as well as revitalizing the skin. Other essential oils for after-sun aromatherapy include lavender and rose. Lavender oil is used medicinally in the treatment of such skin conditions as psoriasis, dermatitis and eczema and to counteract extreme cases of sun damage, including sunstroke and ordinary burns. Rose oil, as well as being antiseptic and soothing, healing and anti-inflammatory, also relieves tension and headaches and is said to act as an aphrodisiac.

BURNING

Sunburn is similar to other burns. Depending on the degree of burn, the skin responds as it does to a scalding from boiling water or hot fat. It becomes red, the blood vessels swell and fragile tissues break. If the burn is superficial, healing begins within two days as fluid is released from the damaged cells and inflamed blood vessels. In more serious cases the fluid forms blisters just under the skin's surface which result in peeling as they burst.

Peeling after sunbathing is caused by burning and cannot be "glued on" again with a moisturiser, which helps to keep dry skin supple, smooth, attractive and young-looking, but cannot reverse burning and peeling.

You can **alleviate the pain of sunburns**. It is advisable to drink lots of cold water, followed by a cool bath or shower which will soothe burnt skin. Next apply a topical remedy to calm inflammation and anaesthetize pain. Moisturising ingredients help the healing process: when the skin is busy manufacturing new cells to repair the damage, these literally "swim" about on the surface of the skin, repairing and renewing damaged areas. This is why water is there in a blister, to facilitate the healing process. Ingredients of value in soothing burns include Aloe vera (Aloe vera gel is often used in the treatment of burns), benzoin, chamomile and witch hazel.

Traditional home-made recipes for sunburn include slices or juice of cucumber placed or patted against affected areas. Juice can be extracted from a whole cucumber (including the skin) by liquidizing it with a few tablespoons of water and straining it through a coffee filter. Strong cold tea is another old-fashioned remedy, as is natural yoghourt, a particularly effective old Greek trick. Cider vinegar is also considered effective, although it stings on application, and so is neat gin.

Other remedies for sunburn pains can be bought from chemists' shops — calamine is a particularly effective old favourite. The most common ingredient in many proprietary brands of sunburn relief is benzocaine or benzocaine derivatives. This is a topical anaesthetic, but a few people are allergic to it and react with a painful rash. In that case, wash off with cool water and avoid other benzocaine preparations to which you will also be allergic. Most such products can be identified by the use of

Fact: sesame seed oil
This is one of the best vegetable oils, screening out about 30% of the sun's ultraviolet rays compared to about 20% of other vegetable oils.

DIY tip: cucumber lotion
30ml cucumber juice
30ml milk
30ml very strong tea
30ml witch hazel
Stir the cucumber juice slowly into the milk, then add the tea and witch hazel, stirring slowly to prevent the milk from curdling. Store in the fridge and shake before use. This has a soothing effect on sunburn.

Chamomile is as soothing and refreshing as ice packs on a hot, sunburnt skin but, unlike ice, chamomile also calms down the inflammation and starts the healing process.

DIY tip: tan erasers
The last odd remnants of a holiday tan can be removed with diluted natural yoghourt, diluted lemon, grape juice or fennel water, or a combination of these. Apply as a compress and leave for at least 20 minutes.

Fact: flying high
The earliest sunscreens were developed during the Second World War as skin protection for pilots of high-flying reconnaissance planes.

"caine" in the name on the ingredients list. Alternatively, make up your own soothing calamine lotion by mixing together 30g of calamine powder and 15g of zinc powder; put them in a small screwtop jar or bottle and add 15ml of glycerine. Shake the bottle thoroughly, adding up to 20 more drops of glycerine to give a creamy lotion. Store it in the refrigerator and shake well before using it over tender, sunburnt spots.

A bad sunburn usually peaks in about 48 hours. Never go back into the sun while you are still suffering from sunburn, it will only make matters worse.

CONTINUED AFTER-SUN CARE

The full lifetime of a tan is around a month, so after-sun care should be more than a quick tonic to be applied after over-exposure. It is essential for keeping your skin smooth, attractive, healthy and young-looking. All the re-moisturising routines should be followed regularly for about a month after you return from holiday, to minimize skin damage and promote healthy new skin.

SUNSCREENS – DO THEY WORK?

One of the most commonly asked questions is "Do beauty preparations really work?" or "Are they worth it?" Even the most expensive suntanning products are quite cheap compared to other beauty preparations, and yes, they really do work. Anyone who has spent a day in strong sun and has forgotten to use a sunscreen can vouch for that. More important is their long-term effect, on the beauty of the skin and particularly on its health. Dermatologists and cosmetic companies agree that UV light is a major factor in skin ageing and cancer; regular use of sunscreens will benefit your skin more than all the "miraculous" ingredients that you may use to repair the damage later on. Instead of burning your skin ruthlessly during the teenage years and turning to expensive creams and unguents in middle age, seeking help in ingredients as bizarre as pregnant mare's urine and extract of edible snails, you would be well advised to spend time and money **protecting your skin against the sun now.** Sunscreens have been the major beauty discovery of this century, and their importance cannot be overrated.

PERFUME

SCENT AND SMELL

CHOOSING A SCENT

WHAT IS PERFUME?

ON THE NOSE

SCENTSATIONAL

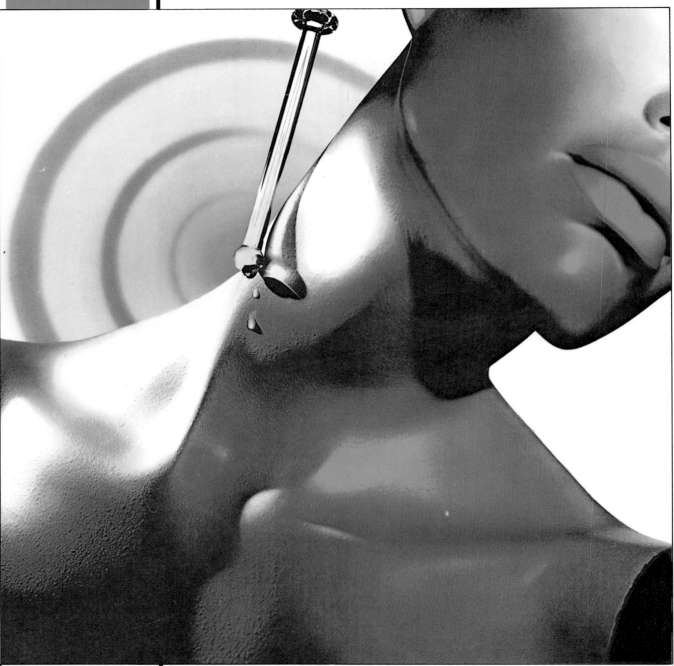

SCENT AND SMELL

CENT PERVADES OUR EVERY WAKING HOUR IN DAILY LIFE. WE surround ourselves with scented toiletries and cosmetics. We clean our homes with fragrant creams and sprays. We wash our clothes in scented detergents and softeners and frantically deodorize the natural smells of our bodies.

And yet for most of us the words "perfume" and "scent" still have a magic ring, denoting an expensive luxury to be worn only on special occasions. Sensual and evocative, there's nothing quite like the joy of spraying a haze of perfume and walking into the haze, or receiving a gift of perfume from a lover or special friend. And that's not new — throughout history perfume made from the finest ingredients has been used to mark momentous events.

PERFUME PSYCHOLOGY – WHAT TURNS YOU ON?

In the animal kingdom scent plays a vital part in survival, and fear and aggression are scented as strongly as sex. But what of the human animal? In what lies perfume's power?

Recently a lot of publicity has been given to pheromones, the chemical "scent signals" used by animals and insects to make sexual contact. In some species the effect is quite dramatic. Male moths, for instance, can track a female a kilometre or so away by her pheromones or "airborne hormones". Several attempts have been made to reproduce pheromones artifically — pig breeders, for example, have experimented with types of spray-on "Instant Boar" in the hope of bringing their sows into heat.

For some years now, the hunt has been on to identify pheromones in human beings. There is a lot of evidence to show that they exist but it seems that they are easily disguised by other smells, such as sweat, tobacco and alcohol. A few years ago a cosmetic company launched a perfume for women and an aftershave for men containing androsterone, the sex hormone contained in the Instant Boar spray. Despite all the wishful thinking and a good deal of publicity, however, the instant chemistry failed to materialize when the products were worn.

It seems that bottling a sexual scent signal for humans is still as elusive as finding an elixir of youth — though some advertisements like to perpetuate the fantasy that your scent can drive the opposite sex wild. This may be an exaggeration but it cannot be denied that scents excite and stimulate the imagination. As Kipling wrote: "scents are surer than sights and sounds to make the heartstrings crack".

HOW DO WE SMELL?

The way we smell an odour is fascinating as it involves our entire being. The signal is triggered by the nose and passed on by the nerves to the brain, from where responses are initiated in the body's organs and fluids. The apparatus which allows

Fact: sign language
When we kiss we are in fact performing a ceremony of greeting by smelling. In many primitive languages the word for kiss or greet is the same as that for smell.

Opposite: *Once in contact with the skin the essences in perfume expand to reveal their full scent. Don't judge a perfume by how it smells on a friend, though, as the scent can be affected by your diet and life-style as well as your skin type.*

us to distinguish smells is located at the top of the nose. Tiny rods project filaments known as the "olfactory hairs" into the nasal mucous membrane. These "hairs" catch odour molecules in the mucous membrane and affect the nerve cells which then send a signal to the brain.

Human beings have about 10 million olfactory nerve cells, while dogs have over twenty times that number. Nevertheless, olfactory sensitivity in human beings is still considerable. The nerve endings of the olfactory cells can be overcome by too strong a smell and prevent the scent being appreciated. Jasmine, for example, is very pleasant in small doses but large quantities can give you a real headache. There is a certain type of briar rose called *Rosa foetida* which has a pleasant enough scent from a distance but a sickening foetid smell close up — hence its name.

Some scents are also said to cause physical injury because of their effect on the nerves. Violet and musk, for example, are reportedly bad for the vocal chords if they are inhaled too closely. This may be an old wives' tale, but it was certainly believed by French scientists of the 19th century.

SMELL, FEELING AND MEMORY

Our sense of smell belongs to our primary instincts and, as such, it is closely associated with our feelings and emotions. When we dislike someone without knowing exactly why just because there is "something about them" which makes us uneasy, it may be because we don't like their smell. Our perception of odour is highly individual and often unpredictable. During pregnancies women quite frequently find they can't stand odours they formerly found attractive. It is hard to say precisely why we like a particular scent as there are many different factors involved in personal selection. But various tests under scientific conditions have produced some interesting results, especially on the psychological reactions of human beings to perfume. Among these is the discovery that perfumes containing a certain percentage of androsterone are usually preferred to those that contain none. It has also been shown that certain moods can be paired with certain odours.

Van Toller has demonstrated that if you associate an unfamiliar odour with a particular emotion, the same emotion can be generated next time you smell that odour. So if you are feeling anxious the first time you smell a particular odour, the next time you smell it, your mood will once again change to anxiety. Perhaps this is why certain people "fall in love" with certain scents — because of the feelings of happiness they associate with them. Perhaps too, it has something to do with the so-called "erotic effect" of certain flowers.

According to Freud, memory helps us to recognize a smell but it doesn't help us to recreate it. You can test this for yourself by trying to bring back a scent by describing it. No matter how many adjectives you use, the actual *scent* will still escape you.

By contrast, the way that odours bring back memories, both good and bad, is almost uncanny. Some smells, especially those to do with food, give us a sense of security — of home, and family and comfort. Others, especially perfumes, are associated with pleasant memories of events, places and, most of all, people. Ask a man why he likes a particular perfume and he will probably tell you it's because it reminds him of a certain woman. And a woman will often stay faithful to a perfume given her by her first love, or one which she associates with some other happy event.

CHOOSING A SCENT

SO HOW CAN YOU FIND THE RIGHT PERFUME? START BY THINKING about *you*. Are you shy, romantic, sexy, glamorous – or all those things in turn? There's no reason why you can't have different perfumes for every occasion, as no single scent will ever suit all your moods.

The most important thing in choosing and buying scent is to try it out first. What smells great on a friend may not suit you at all. In his book *The Psychological Foundations of Perfumery*, the German perfumer, Paul Jellinek, maintains that different ethnic groups have different skin odours, and those affect fragrance. Fair-haired Scandinavian types, according to him, have a skin smell that is similar to rotting leather and decaying butter; redheads have a skin odour like rancid butter mixed with catmint; and brunettes smell like rotting goats!

Be that as it may, what is known is that the smell of the skin changes with life-style and diet, which in turn affects the smell of a perfume. So don't just pick up a bottle and sniff the contents, **always try out a perfume on your own skin.**

When choosing scent, *bear in mind the climate in which it is to be worn. Cool, showery weather will bring out scents, whereas strong, dry heat will make it more difficult to smell. Fragrance is intensified in warm, humid countries.*

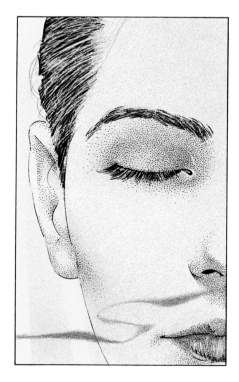

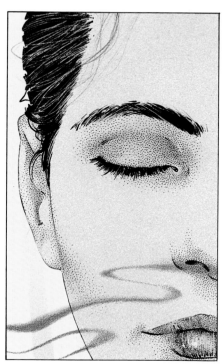

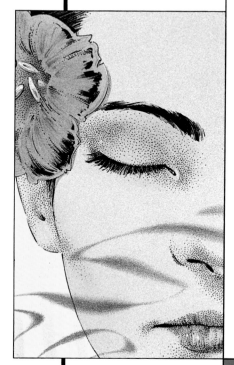

The Body Shops are custom-built for testing and the Perfume Bar provides an excellent introduction to a wide range of different scents. Some perfumes should be left to "develop" on the skin for 10 to 15 minutes, so that the entire range of smells have time to make their presence felt. This is not necessary with Body Shop oil-based perfumes as the aroma unfolds immediately.

Climate also plays an important part in perfume selection. Warm humid atmospheres intensify fragrance, so in tropical climates light, yet lingering fragrances are very popular. Very hot dry climates impair your sense of smell, as the heat dries the mucous membrane in the nose and makes it more difficult to smell acutely. Here it makes sense to use a stronger fragrance. In temperate climates like our own, a sudden shower of rain after a long dry spell stimulates the olfactory sense and almost overpowers it; then you can get "nose fatigue", much the same as when you try to smell too many perfumes in quick succession.

The increasing number of different smells that surround us can also overwhelm our senses, so it is important when choosing a scent to leave the heavily scented atmosphere of the Perfume Bar and wear the perfume in a different environment.

DO'S AND DON'TS FOR BEGINNERS
Don't try too many scents at once — unless you have a trained nose, you will soon become confused. Stick to three or four at a time, testing them on parts of the skin that are as far away as possible from each other.

Perfume can be worn anywhere on the body, but the most effective places are the pulse points: the temples, the nape of the neck, inside the wrists, the crook of the elbow, under the breasts and behind the knees.

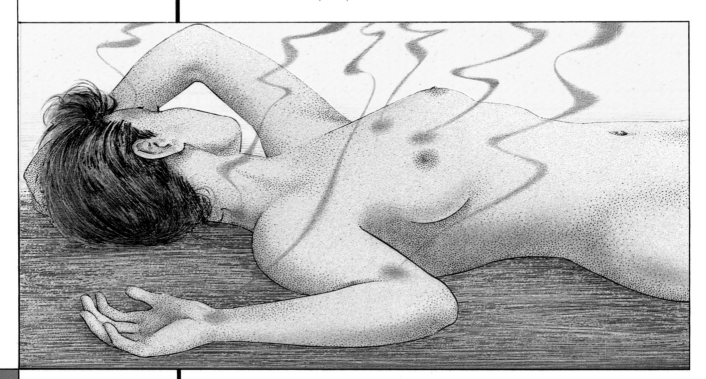

Avoid mixing different scents like strong deodorants and perfume. Any scent takes around six hours to clear from the skin, so if you've just had a bath with a carbolic soap, for instance, this will affect your perfume.

Choose your scent to match your mood and life-style. The light, refreshing scents are best for morning, such as Lemon or Lemon Verbena, or a delicate floral like Rose or Apple Blossom. Keep the heavier "oriental scents", such as Musk, Patchouli, White Musk and Chypre, for evening.

Wear scent wherever you like. Coco Chanel said you should wear it wherever you would like to be kissed! Marilyn Monroe wore it all over herself. Hot spots for perfume are the "pulse points": the inner wrists, the knees, the crooks of the elbows, under the breasts and at the nape of the neck.

Don't keep scent on top of a dressing-table, where it is exposed to direct sunlight or near heat. *Perfume deteriorates when exposed to light, moisture, heat and air, so remember to keep the bottle tightly stoppered when not in use.*

To decant a perfume, first rinse a glass bottle with soapy water, then fill it with half alcohol and half water. Leave it to stand for 24 hours, then rinse again with plenty of fresh water. The Body Shop sell special frosted glass bottles which make ideal perfume containers.

WHAT IS PERFUME?

SO WHAT EXACTLY IS A PERFUME? TO THE LAYMAN, IT IS SIMPLY A sweet-smelling substance. To the perfumer, it is the result of a complicated blending of many different materials. The ingredients of a perfume can be divided into three main groups: essential oils and products isolated from these oils; synthetic materials and natural products of animal origin.

FLOWER POWER

There are three classic methods of separating natural aromatics from raw materials. The first is by *distillation*. This is the most economical way of extracting essential oils and involves literally "steaming out" the fragrance. The second method is by *expression*, which involves squeezing or pressing and is used for removing oils from citrus fruits. The third method is by *extraction*: *enfleurage*, a system of painting lard on to sheets of glass and pressing flower petals into the fat which gradually absorbs their scent; secondly, *maceration*, in which gums and resins are covered with alcohol which is then heated to absorb the perfume, and thirdly, by *using solvents* like petroleum, ether or carbon dioxide to extract the scent of the natural product.

Some floral essences are said to have an aphrodisiac effect. Tuberose has a heavy sweet scent reputed to throw the incautious wearer into a state of sexual frenzy. It is grown in the South of France, Italy and Morocco and is literally worth its weight in gold.

Myth breaker
It's not true that some perfumes are aphrodisiacs. Worn by the right person at the right time, scent can certainly have an erotic effect, but there is no proof that any particular perfume will make you instantly irresistible.

Fact Box
Perfume strengths vary according to the amount of alcohol in them. Perfume or *extrait* contains about 20% perfume (synthetic and natural ingredients) and about 90% alcohol. Eau de Toilette contains even less perfume – between 5 and 12%; the rest is a mixture of alcohol and water. Eau de Cologne is predominantly water, with only a whisper of perfume – between 2 and 6%.
Body shop perfumes are made from perfume blends of synthetic or natural materials. They contain no alcohol or water.

Overleaf Scent is sensual and evocative, pure luxury for the nose. Imagine swimming through a sea of petals.

Another pure luxury in the floral world is rose oil. It comes from the damask rose, grown at the foot of the Balkan mountains. The roses bloom for just 30 days and have to be picked in the early morning as the sun robs the blossoms of their essential oils. The blossoms must be processed quickly, since their fragrance fades with their freshness. Jasmine, in contrast, releases its fragrance long after the flower is picked. It takes about ten tonnes of rose blossoms to produce a single kilo of oil. Lavender is a very popular perfume ingredient, valued for its clean and fresh scent.

Essential oils are not only found in flowers but in leaves and stems, barks, fruits, woods and roots. Patchouli, for example, comes from the leaves of a small plant found in Indonesia and the Philippines. It has a very tenacious odour and was very popular in the 1960s. Vetiver is the aromatic root of a plant which originates from India. There it is used to make sun blinds which, when watered in the sun, give off a scent like violets. Sandalwood comes from trees cultivated in India, Ceylon and Indonesia; it yields an oil with a sweet, mellow scent which blends beautifully in perfume with many other naturals, including rose, lavender and violet. Cedarwood provides another aromatic oil, which was commonly used in the Elizabethan era to scent soaps.

Essential oils provide many of the ingredients used by the perfumer, but an increasing amount are now supplied by synthetics.

SYNTHETIC SUPERSCENTS

Synthetics are often regarded as the poor relations of natural substances and have the reputation of being cheaper and poorer in quality than the real thing. Neither of these is true. Some synthetics now cost more than natural substances and some are in fact better than the natural product.

There are a number of reasons for this: firstly, no two harvests of flowers are ever the same, so maintaining quality is very difficult with natural substances. Not so for synthetics which can always be made to the same level of quality. Also, some natural scents are notoriously disappointing when they are extracted – lilac and hyacinth, for example, rarely smell as good as they do in the garden. In cases like this, artful use of synthetics can actually give a truer rendering of the perfume. Natural ingredients are also very limited in supply and, in the case of animal scents, they involve endangering the species. So it makes sense to use good synthetics, and some of the world's loveliest perfumes include them.

Some synthetics imitate florals or fruits in smell, others have odours that are unknown in nature. They cover many thousands of different types and strengths and make it theoretically possible to produce as many different types of perfume.

As with many great discoveries, success at synthetizing key ingredients has sometimes come about by accident. In the late 19th century, a chemist tried to imitate the scent of violets by mixing oil and other ingredients. The result of his ''brew'' was a failure, so he rinsed out the beaker with strong mineral acids – which suddenly filled the room with the unmistakeable perfume of violets!

ANIMAL MAGIC?

The most controversial perfume ingredients are those extracted from animals. They are diluted with alcohol and today are almost exclusively confined to expensive French perfumes.

LAVENDER

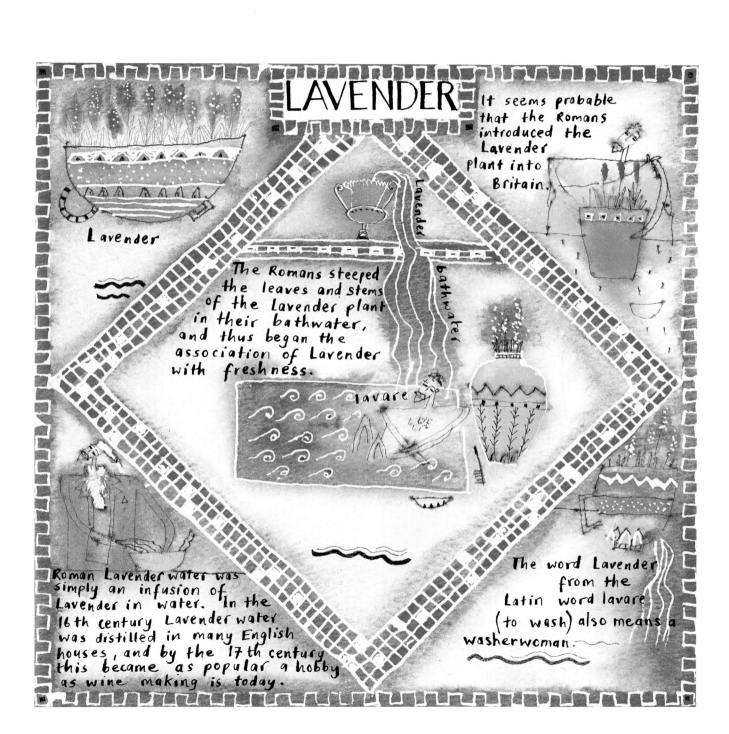

It seems probable that the Romans introduced the Lavender plant into Britain.

Lavender

The Romans steeped the leaves and stems of the Lavender plant in their bathwater, and thus began the association of Lavender with freshness.

Lavender

bathwater

lavare

Roman Lavender water was simply an infusion of Lavender in water. In the 16th century Lavender water was distilled in many English houses, and by the 17th century this became as popular a hobby as wine making is today.

The word Lavender from the Latin word lavare (to wash) also means a washerwoman.

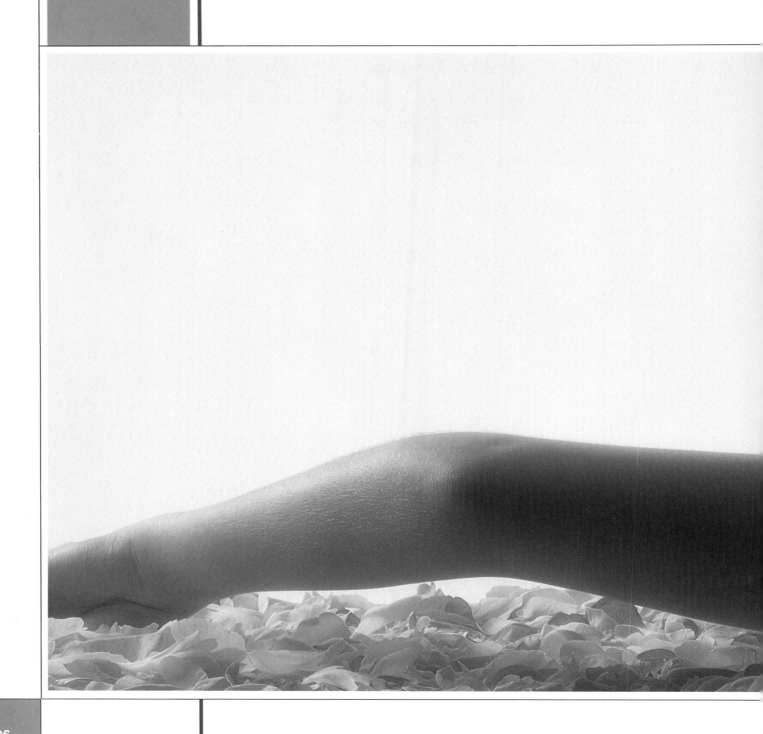

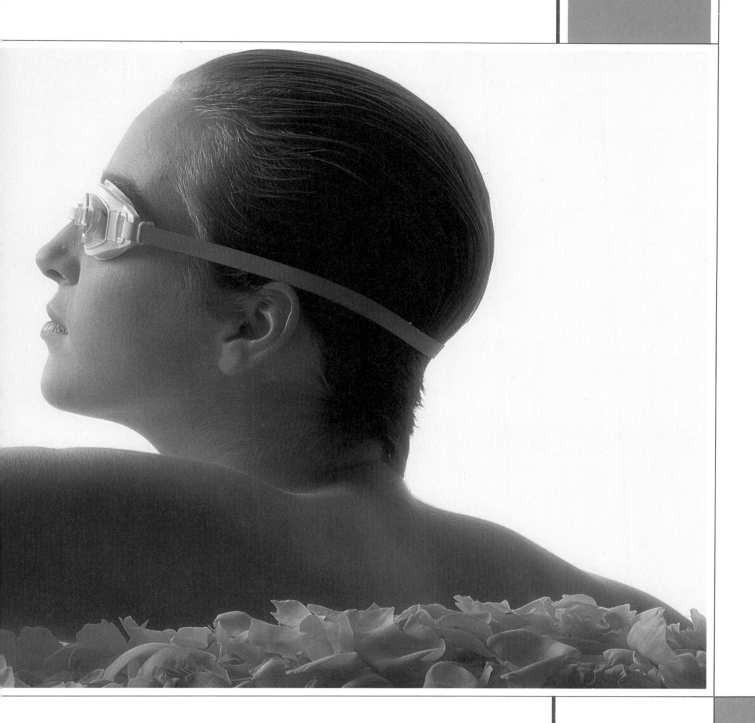

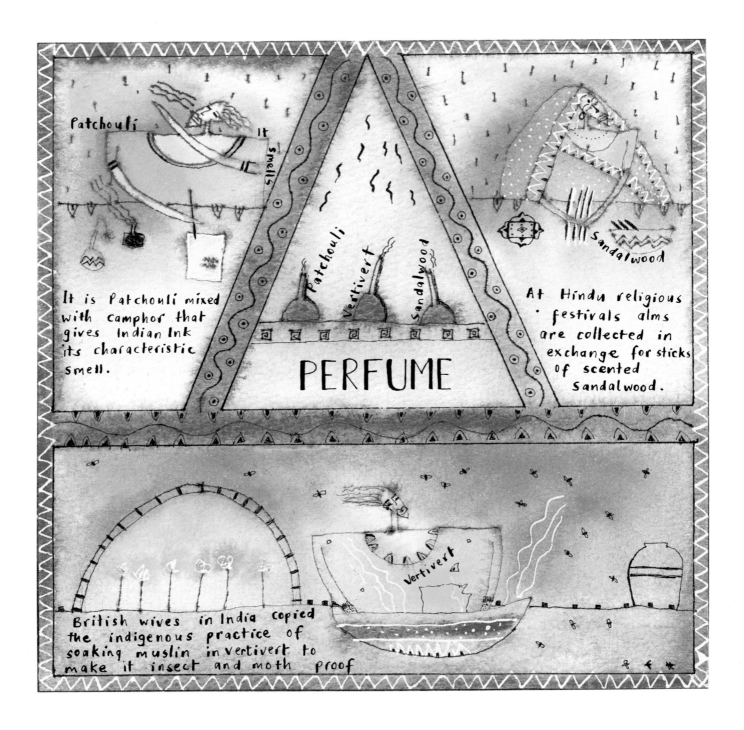

Patchouli

It smells

It is Patchouli mixed with camphor that gives Indian Ink its characteristic smell.

Patchouli   Vertivert   Sandalwood

PERFUME

Sandalwood

At Hindu religious festivals alms are collected in exchange for sticks of scented sandalwood.

Vertivert

British wives in India copied the indigenous practice of soaking muslin in vertivert to make it insect and moth proof

One of the most widely used is civet. 1700 kilos of civet is collected every year, scraped from the sex glands of captive civet cats. This incredibly painful process doesn't kill the animals, however; they are "farmed" for four or five years. The secretion is a soft waxy substance, similar to butter, and in its natural state it has a powerful smell like urine. Once diluted with other ingredients, however, civet gives "punch". In the unlikely event that you should want to buy some, the cost of a kilo equals that of a good second-hand car.

The scent of musk provides the hauntingly sweet "top notes" in several best-selling French perfumes and one or two expensive aftershaves. It is an exceedingly strong scent, however, and a little goes a very long way. Up to 16,000 musk deer are killed every year to provide 320 kilos of musk. Hunted in the mountain crags of Central Asia, amidst the rhododendrons and juniper, this solitary animal is driven towards a decoy in some deep pass or gorge by a line of hunters. One end is closed with a barricade of thorn bushes. When the animals in the area have become trapped, the other end is blocked off and the musk deer are killed. Due to the indiscriminate nature of the process, many deer are killed that yield no "pods", so that although females and young deer do not have the necessary glands they still may not escape the trap. This appalling practice has reduced the musk deer to dangerously low survival levels. Musk is now the most expensive animal product in the world, having replaced ivory. In 1950 it was already worth its weight in gold and, for the price of a kilo today, you could buy a three-bedroomed house. Thankfully, a lot of the musk that is now used in perfume is synthetic – and this does not mean that it is any lower in quality. But sadly synthetic musk still has not displaced natural musk from the top-selling perfumes.

Ambergris, another animal perfume, earned its French name (literally grey amber) because it was originally thought to be a kind of resin. In fact, it comes from the sperm whale and is a result of disease in the poor beast's intestines, caused by the cuttlefish which form part of its diet. It regurgitates these lumps of bile (some 2 metres in diameter) which, due to their high specific gravity, bob about on the surface of the sea until they wash ashore in New Zealand, Australia and elsewhere. The longer they float around in the sun, the more they are worth. Naturally the substance is also found inside slaughtered sperm whales, in about 1 to 10 cases, but then it is often mixed with blood and guts and so is less valuable and much less popular with master perfumers.

Castoreum, taken from the glands of a beaver, initially has very little smell. Its odour develops only when it is dissolved in alcohol, whereupon it becomes so potent as to be positively overpowering. It comes from the lymphatic glands in the beaver's groin, which are then dried in the sun, and today is included in just five French perfumes.

While animal perfumes undoubtedly play an important part in the sex lives of the animals themselves, there is absolutely no scientific proof that wearing them has a similar effect on humans. And given the wealth of good synthetics modern science has made available, we consider the pain and misery caused to the animals completely unjustifiable. We use synthetic ingredients to blend and bouquet perfumes in place of animal ingredients so long as the synthetics themselves have never been tested on animals.

Fact: beauty and cruelty
The civet cat is about the size of a fox, with grey fur and black spots. Each year about 1000 civets are caught and kept in cages for three or four years. The cages are deliberately hot and small, for heat increases the cat's secretions and the cramped space enables the cat to be held while the contents of the gland is scraped off with a small spoon. The secretion is scraped off several times a week. As if this were not enough the "farmers" have learnt that taunting the animal increases the amount of secretion.

Myth breaker
Forget the theory that oils made from synthetic aromatics are not as good as complete naturals – some are even better, and they can replace animal ingredients very satisfactorily.

ON THE NOSE

PERFUME TODAY HAS LARGELY BECOME A PRODUCT FOR THE MASS market. Gone are the days when a perfumer could sit down and follow his own nose, like the famous Francois Coty, who could create a work of art to his own liking, uninhibited by "market pressures".

Some "noses", as perfume blenders are called, have continued the tradition of the solitary artist, however. Men like Edmond Roudnitska who created Femme for Rochas and many of the Dior fragrances, or Jean Paul Guerlain, one of the long family of "noses" who have created an impressive list of highly successful perfumes. Creating a perfume has often been compared to preparing *haute cuisine*, or better still, to composing a piece of music. Balance in music is achieved by the careful harmonization of instruments. In perfume, the "nose" or perfumer also seeks to balance a fragrance by careful harmony of different "notes".

The "top note" of a perfume is the first impression you have of it. The "middle note" comes into play after you have been wearing the perfume long enough for it to dry on your skin and for the different essences to "expand". The bottom or "base note" is the final lingering scent. One or more of these perfume notes may occur in the same scent. A perfume may have a floral top note, for example, and dry down to a woody base note. The main perfume families are the greens (citrusy and sharp), the florals, the orientals, the woody and leather notes, the synthetic aldehydes (which can be floral, woody or oriental) and the chypre notes.

If you think this list sounds rather complicated, consider for a moment the work of the perfumer. While most of us can distinguish a few outstanding scents, the professional must remember literally thousands. He must memorize them as the "building blocks" of his work which includes single essences, complex synthetics, ethereal oils and complete bases. These blocks form the tools of his trade. They are the "fragrance organ" or array of ingredients that he works with. Mixing, measuring, adjusting and rejecting the various ingredients of a single new perfume usually takes from two to four years.

AIR SPRAYS

Owing to the fierce competition in the perfume world today, very few "noses" now work individually. Most are part of large fragrance organizations and their work extends beyond simple perfume to the creation of hundreds of different "fragrance products".

Once we start to think about the fragrance surrounding us in daily life, it may seem as if we live in a scent-soaked atmosphere. For the range of perfumed products is expanding all the time. In fact, though, we are far less perfume-orientated than, say, the 17th century. In those days perfuming was a popular alternative to washing. French high society considered baths to be downright unhealthy, so everything was perfumed – clothes, people, houses, furniture, dogs, horses – the lot.

Today we use perfume less to disguise unpleasant smells than to heighten our awareness of ourselves. Many original perfumes give rise to "product families" of scented soaps, talcum powders, body lotions and bath oils, all with the same fragrance. Then there are the other scented toiletries that we use regularly, such as cleansing milks, face lotions, shampoos and conditioners.

Some scents reinforce the benefits of the product. Take for example, PEPPERMINT OIL. Its high menthol content is stimulative, and can prevent chilblains and even slow hair fall. So whether in a shampoo or a foot cream the two double as scent and active ingredient. ROSEMARY is said to "gladden the spirits" with its pungent smell. Added to shampoo it also makes an effective dandruff chaser.

Citrus fruits have always been known for their bright refreshing smell. LEMON has associations with "cleanliness" for many people and is therefore a popular ingredient in washing-up liquids! ORANGE FLOWER WATER is a well-known tonic for greasy skins. Distilled from neroli oil, it makes a fragrant and refreshing toner for an oily complexion.

Less fragrant perhaps, but no less a part of our "scented surroundings", are household fragrances. These include detergents, polishes and room sprays. Some are contained in aerosols and have a slightly chemical smell. There are much nicer natural alternatives. A few drops of lavender oil added to the household wash, for example, gives linen a lovely clean scent. And pot pourri mixtures with fresh, country-garden scents are much pleasanter than sickly scented room sprays.

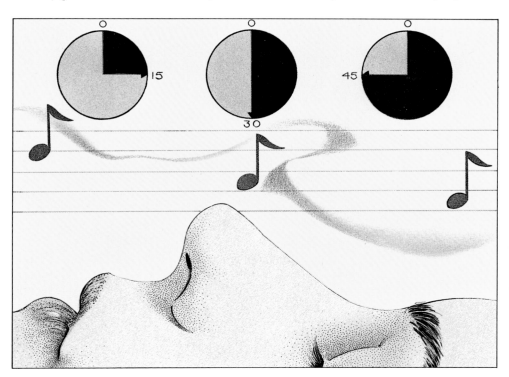

Fact: did you know?
A good sense of smell is very important to doctors when making a diagnosis, because many diseases have their own particular smell. Yellow fever smells like a butcher's shop, typhoid fever like freshly baked bread, plague like apples and measles like freshly plucked feathers!

The composition *of a scent is described in "notes": the "top note" is your first impression on wearing it, the "middle note" becomes noticeable after the perfume has dried on the skin, and the "base note" is the scent which lingers after you have worn it for some time.*

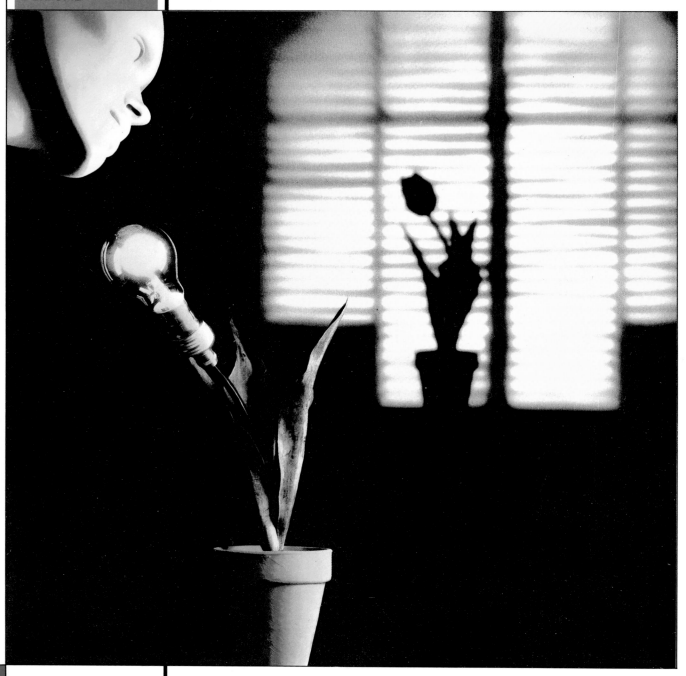

SCENT BOTTLES

Since perfume is a work of art, it has in the past inspired craftsmen in many fields to design suitable containers for scent. Perfume bottles have been made from bronze, gold and precious stones, but the earliest examples also included stone and clay. Alabaster was a particular favourite, because the coolness and density of the material helped prevent evaporation of the perfume. Even today, you are still advised to keep scent in a cool, dark place. With the Roman invention of glass-blowing, glass bottles became popular as scent containers.

Much later on, in the 19th century, scent bottles in England were decorated with silver filigree and mother-of-pearl casings. In Germany, the porcelain industry produced some lovely examples of Meissen perfume bottles, while in France, stunning scent bottles were made in Baccarat glass and in Art Deco designs which gave a whole new look to perfume. Many of these are now collector's items.

Today, it pays to look at what you're purchasing. As any honest perfumer will tell you, when a new perfume is launched, the actual ingredients come very low on the budget. At the top of the list are such items as packaging and promotion.

A French perfumer estimated in 1984 that in a 120ml bottle of toilet water costing around 20 pounds sterling, the major ingredient (say, a concentrated essence) accounted for less than five percent of the purchase price.

SCENTSATIONAL

PERFUME TODAY OWES A GREAT DEAL TO CONTEMPORARY fashion. In this decade, the perfume world has been invaded by "designer fragrances". And yet the first great example of these was Chanel Number 5. Chosen by Coco Chanel to complement her new collection of short, sporty dresses and supremely elegant suits, it was christened "Number 5" simply because this was the scent she liked best from a numbered selection presented to her. It says a lot for Miss Chanel's "nose" that she chose a fragrance that is still one of the top three fragrances.

Nowadays, marketing a perfume is a major business in itself. In fact, advertising and big promotional launches capture most of a perfume's budget. Companies think nothing of jetting hordes of VIPs to exotic surroundings in Morocco or Egypt to promote a new perfume, so continuing a tradition of extravagant showmanship that has become a feature of the contemporary perfume launch. In the 1940s, Carven led the field with a series of Green and White Galas. They presented special "Carven Cups" at smart sporting events, patronized by the *haute monde*, and even sent out special "perfume" cheques to a select number of important people, to be exchanged for Carven perfume. More recently, "Madame de Carven", a new perfume, was launched in a vast pavilion on the outskirts of Paris. Some 500 "celebrities" watched a giant perfume bottle rise from its box amidst a laser-beam display.

True or False?
It's true that perfume deteriorates after about six months once the bottle has been opened, though an unopened glass bottle will keep for about a year. Gradually the perfume changes colour and develops a piney smell. At this point, you should throw it away, but why not wear it around the house or, better still, don't keep it that long – use it.

DIY: scent sampling tip
When smelling a selection of concentrated oils, you can clear your nose for a new scent by smelling the sleeve of your coat – so long as it's wool!

Opposite: *A good way of scenting a room is to dab a little perfume on a light bulb. As the bulb heats up it diffuses the scent of the perfume.*

DIY essential oil
Fill a glass jar with sweet scented herbs or flowers, such as lavender; cover with the most odourless vegetable oil you have, and stopper the jar securely. Leave it in a warm, sunny place for a fortnight or so, then strain off the oil, which should be delicately scented.

Opposite: *The extraction of essential oils for the preparation of perfumes is a sophisticated and costly business. Thousands of tonnes of rose petals are crushed yearly to produce the highly-prized rose oil.*

But for sheer drama, Chanel takes the prize. In 1984, "Coco" was launched in that wonderfully opulent building, the Paris Opera House. A fashion show was held in the sumptuous Long Gallery, which was decorated with thousands of Coco Chanel's favourite white flowers. After this, a champagne dinner was served to 800 guests while an opera singer and an orchestra performed, and a tight-rope walker, dressed in a silver leotard, danced between the balconies on the first floor. Finally, a flock of white doves was released above the heads of the guests. Extravaganzas like these are a calculated attempt to impress a certain selection of the public with the sheer luxury of perfume.

FASHIONS IN PERFUME

Choosing a perfume has a lot to do with an individual's search for identity, and in creating a new fragrance, a great deal of thought is given to what sort of public mood prevails at the time. Revlon's "Charlie" is a stunning example of a success which owed much to thorough market research. In 1973, when Charlie was "born", women were found to be most concerned about careers, self-expression, and shedding the "hearth-and-home" image. Long before they launched their new perfume, Revlon had built a careful image of the ideal "Charlie" woman – around 28 years-old, unmarried, probably working in the creative arts, and intent on developing herself and improving her career. The perfume was a daytime fragrance, chosen to suit a particular life-style, and a great deal of expensive advertising supported the image of a purposeful young woman in trousers and sports jacket, striding down a city street with a small dog in tow.

Five years later, Yves Saint Laurent again captured the mood of the moment with a perfume called "Opium". The very name alarmed some people and intrigued others. It was a time of great media interest in the European drug trade, encouraged by films like *Midnight Express* and *The French Connection*. Saint Laurent himself wrote an article about drugs which curiously coincided with the launch of his new perfume. "Opium" is a rich Oriental fragrance which conjures up an image of exotic mystery, and many a woman fell in love with the name and the image of herself as a Mata Hari, even before she had smelt the scent!

In 1979, Cacharel adroitly captured a new mood. By this time, the pendulum had swung towards femininity, romanticism and nostalgia. In France, Anais is a good old-fashioned Christian name, rather like Annie in Britain; it typifies the kind of girl who likes the softer frillier fashions. "Anais Anais" is a basic floral mixture of white flowers, and it formed a "starting point" for a whole new direction of "white blossom" perfumes for the 80s.

But trends in perfume constantly swing back and forth, and many contemporary scents have a heavier *chypre* note. *Chypre* is the French name for Cyprus, and it is from this island that a 12th century Crusader is said to have first brought *eau de chypre* to Western Europe. Coty created the classic modern "Chypre" in 1917, a perfume enhanced by spice oils of cinnamon, clove, coriander, basil and thyme. From this, other spicy blends developed, including Guerlain's "Mitsouko", Rochas' "Femme" and "Miss Dior". Chanel's latest perfume, "Coco", is a *chypre* base with a leather note.

Creating a new perfume is now a highly competitive business. New synthetic materials are patented and sell at high prices. Formulas are jealously guarded and so

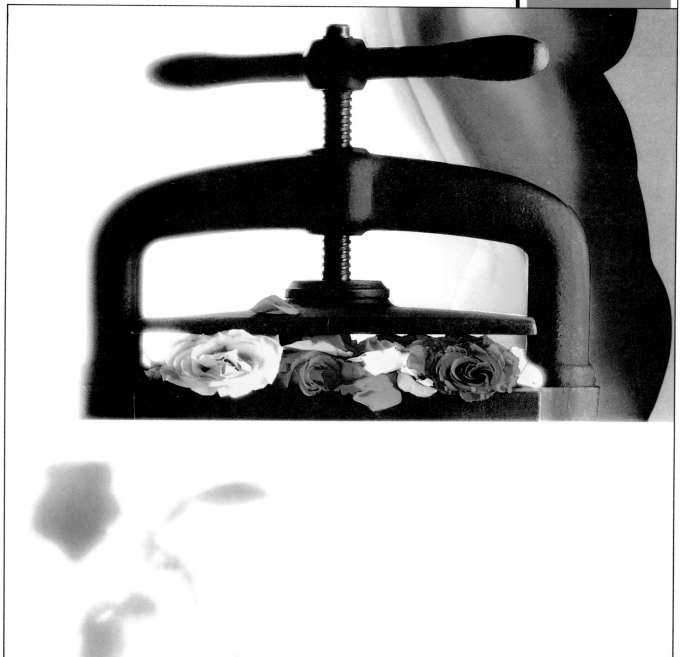

Myth-breaker: scent spots
Where's the best place to apply perfume – behind the ears? Absolutely not! Surprisingly, women perspire a lot in that area and nothing kills the desired effect faster than sweat.

are new manufacturing techniques. Some perfumers feel that the mass market approach has taken the originality out of perfumery. But this isn't always the case. There are still those who distil oils into relatively simple scents and continue to produce plain classics, like lavender, rose and jasmine.

In the end, though, no matter how wonderful the blending, how first-class the ingredients or how clever the advertising or promotion, a perfume is judged above all else on its performance. A perfume only rates as "good" when the wearer likes it and it pleases the people around her.

Perfume prices are often very inflated, but a fine fragrance can be very seductive and, like all luxuries, it's worth paying the price if it makes you happy. As with any beauty care, however, there is much to be said for beginning with the basics and deciding, without the market hype, what really suits *you* best. Remember, a rose by any other name will always smell as sweet.

BODY SHOPS AROUND THE WORLD

ENGLAND

8 High Street
Aylesbury
Bucks HP20 1SQ

Unit 39-41
The Eastgate Centre
Basildon
Essex SS14 1XB

8 Green Street
Bath BA1 2JY
Avon

37 New Street
Birmingham
West Midlands

5 North Western Arcade
Birmingham B2 5LH
West Midlands

19 High Street
Bognor Regis PO21 1RJ
West Sussex

98 Old Christchurch Road
Bournemouth BH1 1LR
Hants

41/43 North Street
Brighton BN1 1RH
East Sussex

33/33a Queens Road
Bristol BS8 1QG
Avon

20 Westmoreland Centre
Bromley BR1 1DR
Kent

6 Rose Crescent
Cambridge CR2 3LL
Cambs

20 Burgate
Canterbury CT1 2HG
Kent

41 Regent Arcade
Cheltenham GL50 1JZ
Glos

9 Paddock Row
Grosvenor Precinct
Chester CH1 1ED
Cheshire

34/35 East Street
Chichester PO19 1HS
West Sussex

22 Broad Walk
Crawley
West Sussex RH10 1HQ

4 Rothschild House
The Whitgift Centre
Croydon
Surrey CR0 0XB

1037 The Whitgift Centre
Croydon CR0 1UU
Surrey

32 Green Lane
Derby DE1 1RX
Derbyshire

21 Elvet Bridge
Durham DA1 3AA
Durham

21 Guild Hall Centre
Exeter EX4 3H4
Devon

61/62 Central Arcade
Great Yarmouth NR30 2NU
Norfolk

181 High Street
Guildford GU1 3AW
Surrey

11-15 St Anns Road
Harrow
Middlesex HA1 1LQ

6 Middle Street
Horsham RH12 1NW
West Sussex

91 George Street
Hove BN3 3YE
East Sussex

7-9 The Walk
Ipswich IP1 1EA
Suffolk

6/8 Thames Street
Kingston upon Thames
SL4 1EA
Surrey

9 Trinity Street Arcade
Leeds LS1 6QN
Yorks

9 Cheapside
Leicester LE1 5E6
Leics

5a Bold Street
Liverpool L1 4DJ
Merseyside

1a White Hart Lane
Barnes
London SW13 0PX

22/23 Cheapside
London EC2V 6AB

Unit 13
The Market
Covent Garden
London WC2E 8RB

32/34 Great Marlborough
Street
London W1V 1HA

62 Gayton Road
Hampstead
London NW3 1TU

7 Upper Street
Islington
London N1 0PQ

203 Kensington High Street
London W8 6BA

54 Kings Road
London SW3 4UD

65 Kings Road
London SW3 4NT

The Floral Centre
18-26 Long Acre
London WC2E 9LD

194 Portobello Road
London W11 1LA

113 Victoria Street
London SW1E 6RA

Unit 345/346
Dukes Walk
Stoneborough Centre
Maidstone ME15 6AS
Kent

28 The Arndale Centre
Manchester
Lancs M4 2HU

Royal Exchange Shopping
Centre
Cross Street
Manchester M2 7DB

130 Grainger Street
Newcastle upon Tyne NE1 5AF
Tyne & Wear

14 Sidgate
Newcastle-upon-Tyne NE1 7XF
Tyne & Wear

18 Peacock Way
Northampton NN1 2DJ
Northants

8 Castle Street
Norwich NR2 1PD
Norfolk

8 Bridlesmith Gate
Nottingham NG1 2GS
Notts

125 High Street
Oxford OX1 4DF
Oxon

Unit 59
Queensgate Centre
Peterborough PE1 1NH
Cambs

71 The Arndale Centre
Poole
Dorset BH15 2SY

15 Union Street
Reading RG1 1EU
Berks

14 South Street
Romford RM1 1RH
Essex

76 Mardol
Shrewsbury SY1 1PZ
Salop

81a St Peter's Street
St Albans AL1 3EG
Herts

16 Bargate
Southampton SO1 0AD
Hants

Unit 2
75 Union Street
Torquay
Devon TQ1 3DA

18 Chapel Place
Tunbridge Wells TN1 1YQ
Kent

78 Cathedral Walk
The Ridings
Wakefield WF1 1YD
Yorks

31 Peascod Street
Windsor SL4 1EA
Berks

Unit 6 Crown Passage
Broad Street
Worcester WR1 3LX
Worcs

129 Montague Street
Worthing BN11 3BP
West Sussex

14 The Coppergate
York

WALES
Tivoli Gardens
St Davids Centre
Cardiff

SCOTLAND
St Nicholas Centre
St Nicholas Street
Aberdeen AB1 1HW

Unit 11
The Waverley Market
Edinburgh EH1 1BQ

42 Argyll Arcade
Glasgow G2 8AG

NORTHERN IRELAND
10 Castle Lane
Belfast BT1 5DA

CHANNEL ISLANDS
11 Halkett Street
St Helier
Jersey

16 Charing Cross
St Helier
Jersey

EIRE
86 Patrick Street
Cork
Co Cork

Powerscourt Town House
Centre
South William Street
Dublin 2

BELGIUM
Chaussee D'Ixelles 90
Brussels

DENMARK
City Arkaden
Østergade 32
1100 Copenhagen K

FINLAND
Sibeliuksenk. 13
13100 Hameenlinna

100 Roobertink 1
00120 Helsinki

Sornaisten Metrosema
00500 Helsinki

Sopet Tavaratalo
00400 Jarvepaa

Keskuskatu 35
48100 Kotka

Kauppalank 6
45100 Kouvola

Aleksanterink 9
15110 Lahti

Torikatu 15
76100 Pieksamaki

Kauppakatu 9
26100 Rauma

Turuntie 7
24100 Salo

Kuninkaank 28
33100 Tampere

Kristiinank 9
20100 Turku

Kauppapuistikko 14
65100 Vaasa

Neilikkatie 4
01300 Vantaa

FRANCE
11 Rue d'Assas
75006 Paris

GERMANY
Freisenwall
14 Am Rudolf Platz
Cologne

7 Friedrick Ebert Anlage
69 Heidelberg

Aegidiistrasse 3
3300 Munster

Uhlamd Strasse 165
D 1000
West Berlin 15

GREECE
Evergreen Shopping Land
1 Kolokotroni Str.
Kifissia
Athens

Kanari 8 Kolonaki
Athens

Vas Konstantinou 36
Halandri
Athens

Pantheon Kriari
Chania
Crete

HOLLAND
Kalverstraat 202
Amsterdam

Halstraat 27
4811 HV Breda

Eastwick Trading B.V.
Nijverheidswers 34
1402 BW Bussum

Nieuve Rijn 6
Leiden

ICELAND
Laugavegur 66
101 Reykjavik

ITALY
Via Natta
Como

Poethe SRL
26 Via Avogadro
Turin

Firanka Italiana SRL
Via Pacini 51
Catania
Sicily

NORWAY
Hegdehaugsvn 24
0352 Oslo 3

SWEDEN
Kingsgatan 25
411 19 Gothenburg

St Petri Kyrkogata 7
222 21 Lund

Södra Forstadsgatan 68
214 20 Malmö

Köpmannavaruhuset Linden
Drottninggatan
602 25 Norrköping

Storatorget 14
Örebro

Traktoren
Prästgata 24
Östersund

Box 2127
10314 Stockholm

Tinghuset
Östra Langgatan 23
852 36 Sundsvall

Kungsgatan 14
461 31 Trollhättan

Fenixhuset
Svartbecksgatan 6
751 48 Uppsala

Stora Gatan 44c
722 12 Västeras

SWITZERLAND
Preyergasse 8
8001 Zurich

Stadelhoferstrasse 22
8001 Zurich

CYPRUS
Stelmaria Court
220 Makarios Avenue
Limassol

1B Koumanoudi Street
(off Stassicratous Street)
Nicosia

UNITED ARAB EMIRATES
50 Bahrain Commercial Complex
P.O. Box 32165
Manama
Bahrain

Al Qubaisi Building
Hamdan Street
P.O. Box 2333
Abu Dhabi

P.O. Box 12386
Dubai

MALAYSIA
G-56 Ground Floor
Plaza Yow Chuan
Jln Tun Razak
Kuala Lumpur

SINGAPORE
605B Macpherson Road
Citimac Industrial Complex
Hex 03-10

HONG KONG
B1 Shop 18C
Landmark
Des Voeux Road
Central Hong Kong

G/F & I/F D'Aguilar Place
D'Aguilar Street
Central Hong Kong

G/F Room 14
Excelsior Shopping Centre
Causeway Bay

39 Chung Hum Kok Road
Chung Hum Kok

212 Ocean Centre
Canton Road
Tsimshatsui
Kowloon

G/F No. 33 Carnarvon Road
Tsimshatsui
Kowloon

AUSTRALIA
Shop 45
Bondi Junction Plaza
Bondi Junction
N.S.W. 2022

Shop 7a
Pacific Fair Shopping Centre
Broadbeach
Queensland 4217

234 Collins Street
Melbourne 3000

State Bank Galleria
Little Collins Street
Melbourne

3 Chadstone Shopping Centre
Dandenong Road
Melbourne

Church Street
Brighton
Melbourne 3186

7 Bernard Street
Mount Waverley
3149 Melbourne

Moresise PTY
The Body Shop
Tweed City Shopping Centre
Tweed Heads
New South Wales

Cinema City Arcade
Barrack Street
Perth

CANADA
225 7th Avenue S.W.
Unit 325
Scotia Fashion Centre
Calgary
Alberta T2B 2W3

21 Micmac Boulevard
MicMac Mall
Dartmouth
Nova Scotia B3A 4N3

Store No. 370
51 Avenue & 111st
Southgate Mall
Edmonton
Alberta T6H 4M8

West Edmonton Mall
U101, 900, 9707-110th Street
Edmonton
Alberta TK5 2L9

939 Lawrence Avenue E
Don Mills Centre
Don Mills
Ontario M3C 1P8

5640 Spring Garden Road
Spring Garden Place
Halifax B3J 3M7
Nova Scotia

Limeridge Mall
999 Upper Wentworth Street
Hamilton
Ontario L8A 4W5

Orchard Park Shopping Centre
2271 Harvey Avenue N
Kelowna
British Columbia V1Y 6H2

945 Gardiners Road
Cataraqui Town Centre
Kingston
Ontario K7M 7H4

Masonville Place
London
Ontario

785 Wonderland Road
Westmount Mall
London
Ontario N6K 1M6

100 City Centre Dr
Unit A41
Square One Shopping Centre
Mississauga
Ontario L5B 2C9

50 Rideau Street
Unit No. 366
The Rideau Centre
Ottawa
Ontario K1N 9JT

1200 St Laurent Street
St Laurent Shopping Centre
Ottawa
Ontario K1K 3B8

Pickering Town Centre
1355 Kingston Road
Pickering
Ontario L1V 1B8

104th & 152nd Street
Unit #2693
Guildford Mall
Surrey
British Columbia V3R 7C1

1 Dundas Street West
Box 55
Toronto Eaton Centre
Toronto
Ontario M5G 1Z3

101 Yorkville Avenue
Toronto
Ontario M5R 1C1

1st Canadian Place
Store 33
P.O. Box 472
Toronto
Ontario M5X 1E4

650 West 41st Avenue
Oakridge Shopping Centre
Unit No. 437
Vancouver
British Columbia V5Z 2M9

3102 C Shelbourne Street
Hillside Shopping Centre
Unit No. 49
Victoria
British Columbia

100 Park Royal
Unit No. 2086
Park Royal Shopping Centre
West Vancouver
British Columbia V7V 3N6

234 Donald Street #63
Eaton Place
Winnipeg
Manitoba R3C 1M8

St Vital Shopping Centre
Unit C4
86-1225 St Marys Road
Winnipeg
Manitoba R2M 5E5

BAHAMAS
Unit 3
Gleniston Gardens Shopping
Plaza
Nassau

BODY SHOP PRODUCTS

SOAPS
Coconut Milk Soap
Elizabethan Wash-Balls
   (*Rose, Spice*)
Glycerine Fruit Soaps
   (*Apple, Apricot, Lemon, Mandarin*)
Glycerine with Almond Soap
Goat's Milk with Honey Soap
Guest Soap
   (*Apple, Lemon*)
Jojoba Oil Soap
Lily Milk Soap
Orchid Oil Soap
Sauna Soap
   (*Apple, Lemon*)
Vitamin E Soap

FACIAL CLEANSERS
Cucumber Cleansing Milk
Glycerine and Oat Facial Lather
Honeyed Beeswax, Almond and Jojoba Oil
   Cleanser
Milk Protein Cleansing Bar
Orchid Oil Cleansing Milk
Pineapple Facial Wash
Viennese Chalk Facial Wash

FACIAL TONERS
Elderflower Water
Honey Water
Orange Flower Water
White Grape Skin Tonic

FACIAL CREAMS
Aloe Vera Moisture Cream
Carrot Moisture Cream
Jojoba Oil Moisture Cream
Rich Night Cream with Vitamin E
Vitamin E Day Cream

FACIAL SPECIALS
Elderflower Eye Gel
Honey and Oat Scrub Mask
Japanese Washing Grains
Lip Balm
   (*Apricot, Kiwi Fruit, Morello Cherry*)
Neck Gel
Sage and Comfrey Open Pore Cream

HAIR SHAMPOOS
Chamomile Powder Shampoo
Chamomile Shampoo
Coconut Oil Shampoo

Frequency Wash Shampoo
Henna Cream Shampoo
Jojoba Oil Shampoo
Ice Blue Shampoo
Orange Spice Shampoo
Rosemary Shampoo
Seaweed and Birch Shampoo

HAIR TREATMENT PRODUCTS
Aromatherapy Scalp Oil
Chamomile Flower Hair Rinse
Elderberry Conditioner
Hair Gel (*Coconut Oil*)
Hair Salad
Henna Treatment Wax
Protein Cream Rinse
Slick
Soft Style

HERBAL HAIR COLOURS
Blonde
Brown
Egyptian Henna
Extra Red
Rich Red

BATH OILS AND SALTS
Bath Oil
   (*Herb, Musk, Rose*)
Bath Oil Beads
   (*Apple, Lemon, Rose, Strawberry*)
Bath Oil Powder
   (*various fragrances*)
Bath Salts
   (*Apple, French Vanilla, Lemon, Tea Rose*)
Foaming Bath Oil
   (*Herb, Musk, Rose*)
Herb Body Shampoo/Shower Gel
Milk Bath
Orange Cream Bath Oil
Raspberry Ripple Bathing Bubbles
Strawberry Body Shampoo

TALCUM POWDERS AND DEODORANTS
Talcum Powders
   (*Samarkand, Tea Rose*)
Body Shop Deodorant (*roll-on*)

HAND AND BODY LOTIONS AND
   CREAMS
Aloe Gel
Aloe Heat Lotion
Aloe Lotion

Body Massage Oil
Cocoa-Butter Hand and Body Lotion
Cocoa-Butter Suntan Lotion
Glycerine and Rosewater Lotion with
   Vitamin E
Hawthorn Hand Cream
PABA Sunscreen
Peppermint Foot Lotion
Rich Massage Lotion
Sunscreen
Tanning Butter

AROMATHERAPY OILS
Bath Oils
   (*Relaxing, Refreshing, Athletic*)
Body Oils
   (*unscented or scented with Perfume Oils*)
Essential Oils
   (*Chamomile, Eucalyptus, Lavender, Neroli, Peppermint, Rose Absolute, Tangerine*)
Massage Lotions
   (*Relaxing, Refreshing, Athletic*)
Massage Oils
   (*Relaxing, Refreshing, Athletic*)

PERFUME OILS
Concentrates, containing no alcohol:
   (*Al Sabah, Amber, Apple Blossom, Chypre, Coconut, Frangipani, Frankincense, Freesia, Herb, Honeysuckle, Lavender, Lemon, Lemon Verbena, Lilac, Lotus, Moss, Muguet, Musk, Patchouli, Rose, Strawberry, Tea Rose, Vetiver, Woody Sandalwood*)
Body Shop Copy Cats:
   Annie (*Anais-Anais type*)
   L'aird (*L'Air-du-Temps type*)
   Samarkand (*Paco-Rabane type*)
   Rome (*Paris type*)
Scentsationals:
   Summer Dew
   White Musk
   Winter Dew

NATURAL OILS
Anti-Cellulite Oil
Apricot Kernel Oil
Carrot Facial Oil
Coconut Suntan Oil
Jojoba Oil
Sweet Almond Oil
Wheatgerm Oil

HERBS AND POT POURRIS
Lavender Flowers
English Garden Pot Pourri
Rose Pot Pourri

MOSTLY FOR MEN
Shaving: Elizabethan Wash Balls (*Spice*)
    Sandalwood Shaving Cream
After Shaves: Jamaica (*geranium, lavender,*
    bergamot, sage)
    Raffles (*citrus flower, fruits,*
    musk)
    Samarkand
Talcum Powder: Samarkand
Hair Shampoo: Ice Blue Shampoo
Creams: Aloe Vera Moisture Cream

SPECIALITIES AND ACCESSORIES
Blackhead Removers
Body Buddies (*massage mitts*)

Coolpacs
Cosmetic Brush Sets
Emery Boards
Essential Balm
Eye Crayon Sharpeners
Eye Crayons, Jumbo
    (*blue, black, grey, green*)
Eyelash Curlers
Hair Bends
Henna Application Brushes, Caps and Gloves
Herb Sleep Pillows
Herb Snore Pillows
Leg Wax
Loofahs and Loofah Mitts
Make-up Remover Pads
Linen Drawer Sachets
    (*Vetiver, Sandalwood*)
Mascara
    (*black, azure, black/brown*)
Papier Poudre

Pumice Stones
Sponges (*natural Mediterranean Sea*
    sponges, 3 and 5cm for application and
    cleansing of make-up, 10 and 15cm for
    baths and showers)
Towelling Headbands

GIFT ITEMS
Amphora Pots
Fandangles (*scented fabric on ropes*)
Glass Perfume Bottles
Skin Towels & Skin Sponges (*for exfoliation*)
Travel Pack, Clear Plastic Wallet
    (*60ml bottles of Coconut Oil Shampoo,*
    Cucumber Cleansing Milk, Cocoa-Butter
    Hand and Body Lotion)
Weekender, Clear Plastic Wallet
    (*60ml bottles of Orchid Oil Cleansing Milk,*
    Elderflower Water and Glycerine and
    Rosewater with Vitamin E)

ACKNOWLEDGEMENTS

Copy editor: Lizzie Boyd
Designer: David Fordham
Design assistant: Carol McCleeve
Photographs: Charlie Stebbings
Full page theme illustrations: Bina Dhanani
All other illustrations: Jon Geary
Photographs hand tinted: Helena Rucinska-Zakrzewska

INDEX